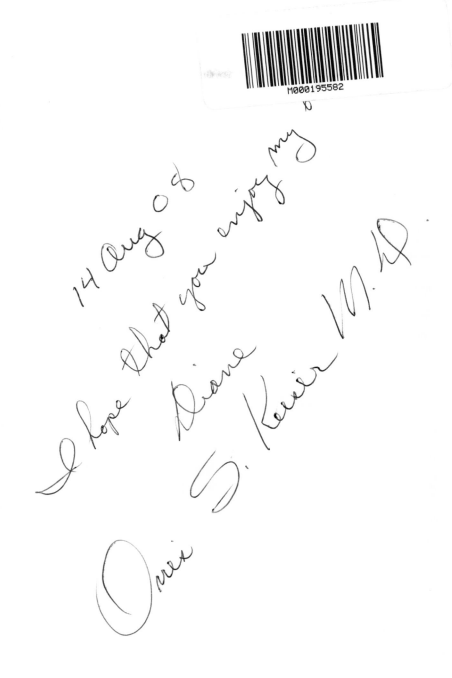

14 Aug 08

I hope that you enjoy my

Diane

S. Keider M.D.

Once

How Can I Help You?

How Can I Help You?

From Family Doctor
to Ship's Physician

Orris S. Keiser, M.D.

VANTAGE PRESS
New York

Published by Vantage Press, Inc.
419 Park Ave. South, New York, NY 10016

Manufactured in the United States of America
ISBN: 0-533-15211-9

Library of Congress Catalog Card No.: 2005903014

0 9 8 7 6 5 4 3 2 1

This book is dedicated to my six grandchildren. It has been written with the hope that they will learn more about their heritage and have a deeper understanding of the life that I have lived.

Contents

1. The Early Years   1
2. Starting Out   27
3. Thirty Years in Wisconsin   42
4. Sailing   102
5. In Conclusion   169

Postscript   179

How Can I Help You?

1

The Early Years

It was a dark and stormy night and I was sleeping restlessly. Somewhere around four A.M. I began to reflect on my life and think about the future. I was seventy-six years old thinking seriously about retiring. Well, maybe not until next year. The next question was, what should I do in retirement? I thought about writing a book, one that would cover my life and the practice of medicine over the last fifty years. With these thoughts in mind, I jumped out of bed and began to jot down some of the highlights of my life, some of the heartaches, and yes even some of the humorous things that have happened. Before I knew it, two hours had gone by and my wife of nearly fifty-five years was out of bed. I began to enthusiastically relate to her the things that I had been thinking. Her reply was, "Now don't get senile on me. That would really be living in the past."

The more I thought about my idea, and the more I thought about her statement, the more I began to think there's nothing better a person can do than think about their past—particularly in my case, when I have so much of it. As for the future of my life, at this point it's uncertain and it surely may be limited.

Before I could start my book, I needed a title. What about, *Fifty Years Practicing Medicine,* or *Medicine Then and Now,* or even *Medicine Now and Then?* Not good. Then

I began to wonder, what my goals have been during these fifty years. What one statement or question have I repeatedly used as I would sit down with a patient? It would either be, "What can I do for you?" or "How can I help you?" *How can I help you?*—that was really what it was all about. So, now with a title here goes!

I was born in Monroe, Michigan, on May 17, 1927. My father was the pastor of the local Seventh-Day Adventist Church. My mother really wanted to be a nurse. She had started out in nursing school but did not complete all of the requirements to become a Registered Nurse. She cut her education short and married my dad. My father did not believe that he was called on by God to become a minister; he felt he had been appointed by his father, although he believed that God had used him to help others.

My father was the youngest in a large family. His mother died of pulmonary tuberculosis when he was just eighteen months old. My grandfather owned a large brick and tile manufacturing plant in Prattville, Michigan. He didn't believe in child labor—but he believed in his children laboring. I can remember my father saying, "When I was growing up and when I was your age, I would sit on a stool all day long. My feet would not even touch the floor and I would be sitting there cutting tile."

My father had an older brother, Ernie, who was studying to be a minister. During his summer vacations, Ernie worked in my grandfather's tile plant and brickyard. His clothing got caught in a large pulley one day at work; and he was crushed to death against one of the walls of the plant. My grandfather was called to the plant, and after seeing what had happened, he never set foot in that building again. He closed the operation and he took up farming.

When Ernie died my father was in high school. He wasn't sure what he wanted to do with his education or with his life, but he was leaning toward becoming a chiropractor. There was no question in my grandfather's mind that logically my father was the one to take Ernie's place and become the family minister.

My father spent his college days in southern Michigan while my mother was in nursing school in the Chicago area. My father has recounted how he saved his money until he had enough to buy my mother a box of candy. His roommate offered to mail the box to her, but instead he opened it and ate all the candy. Then he placed an old, used shoe-brush into the box, rewrapped it, and mailed it to my mother. My parents still managed to fall in love, and were married in 1918.

At the time of my birth I had three sisters. One was nearly five years old. Another was more than six years old, and the oldest was a little more than eight years old. With my sisters close in age and also in spirit, I frequently felt like an only child as I was growing up. The Adventist denomination back then moved its ministers to new positions frequently. When I was around two years of age the whole family moved to Michigan. First we moved to Owosso, from there we moved to Pontiac, where I attended kindergarten, and then we went to Kalamazoo, where I attended first grade. My father was then transferred to a church in Wisconsin, and our family moved. This is where I really feel I did my growing up. Grades two through seven were in Eau Claire. I was a good student during the period, and I was rather shy. The worst thing that I can remember doing was writing my initials almost everywhere with the initials of Iris Miller. She was a girl in my class who I thought was pretty nice. Of course Iris Miller was I.M. and my initials were O.K., so I thought it was pretty smart to write IM OK on things.

The most embarrassing moment that I can remember

happened on a Saturday morning in church. I had a female Boston terrier named Boots because she had white feet. She was the light of my life. She was my constant companion. Every morning I would let her out into the yard. After playing with her and feeding her, I would put her back into the house before going out. However, on this day it was very warm, and she never strayed from our yard when she was left alone, so I didn't put her in the house like I was supposed to do. We went to our church, which was three or four blocks from our home. It was before the invention of air-conditioning, and they had left the front door open to let some of the warm air out, and let the breeze in. My father was right in the middle of his eloquent sermon and my dog walked in. The first thing she saw was my father on the platform. She ran down the aisle and up onto the platform, and stood there, wagging her whole body. She had hardly any tail, and when she was happy everything moved! Needless to say, my father wasn't happy at all. He stopped his sermon right then and there, looked down to where I was sitting and sternly said, "Orris Keiser, you come up here, you get your dog and take her home. And see to it that she is properly secured!" I was very embarrassed and red in the face. With much difficulty, I went up to the platform, picked Boots up, carried her out of the church, and then ran all the way at full speed home. Needless to say, I didn't return to church that day.

My father's hobby was growing flowers—well, vegetables also, but there was nothing as beautiful as the dahlias and gladiolus that adorned our yard. He enjoyed developing new varieties of dahlias, which he would register and name. We had a lot of flowers. When there were more flowers than we could use, or that he could give to the neighbors, he encouraged me to go door-to-door to sell them. All the money that came in from this enterprise was mine, and

I could use it any way that I wished. This was how I was able to buy my first pair of skis. Every kid in Eau Claire skied. In fact, the local grade school had a ski scaffold in the school yard that you could jump from. I'd seen kids go through the air seventy or eighty feet from this ski scaffold. Oh, how I envied them. So I decided to use flower money to buy a new pair of skis. They were maple, and had no fancy bindings, just a leather half circle that I put my shoes into because I didn't have any ski boots. I cut rubber bands out from an old inner tube, and used them to keep my feet in place. We lived on a hillside, and I built a ski jump on it from snow and practiced jumping on it for a week or two, until I could jump eight or ten feet. Then I figured I was ready to go to the real ski hill.

I climbed the scaffold and put on my skis, but then I began to feel a little reluctant about going down the hill. With all my buddies standing around, I couldn't walk down the ski scaffold, so off I went. I had no problem getting down to the bottom of the scaffold, but the flying through the air wasn't what I had expected, and when I contacted the ground, I think my skis were probably going sideways. I rolled the rest of the way down the hill. I had no broken bones; my skis did come off, just like the skis with fancy bindings. I'll tell you one thing—it was a long, long time before I tried that hill again!

I also used flower money to purchase my first bicycle. Our neighbor usually rode a bike to work, but during this winter the weather was more severe than usual, so he purchased a car and put his bike up for sale. It cost fifteen dollars for a bike that looked like new, was bright red, and had balloon tires—and there were two feet of snow on the ground! The snow didn't stop me from learning. My riding was all indoors. It was largely between the living room and the kitchen. As I look back on this, I really don't know how my mother was able to stand that type of activity!

My Grandmother Keiser was dead long before I was born so I have no memories of her. My Grandfather Keiser died when I was four years old and my only memory of him was when we visited him in the hospital. He was dying of cancer of the prostate. I also remember his funeral. My aunt Inez lived close by Grandpa Keiser's place and during his funeral, we stayed at her house. The funeral was held in her parlor, and Grandpa was downstairs in his coffin. I was supposed to stay upstairs, but I didn't. I wanted to be down where all the action was.

I have many fond memories of my mother's parents, Grandma and Grandpa Boist. Grandpa Boist lived until I was thirteen and we frequently went to visit him on his farm. He had an early model Ford that needed to be cranked in order to start. During the winter, my grandfather would put down the side curtains and we would snuggle down in the back seat under a buffalo robe, and off we would go.

Our visits, however, were more often in the summer. There were always chickens running around the farmyard. Near the backdoor was a block of wood with two nails partially pounded into the end of it. When Grandma decided that we were going to have chicken dinner, she would catch a chicken by the feet and she would place the neck between the two nails. With one quick blow of the hatchet, the head was off. The chicken would run around in circles for a while before it dropped dead. I used to think the whole process was pretty amazing!

Grandpa didn't own a tractor. He did his plowing and other farm work with horses. Occasionally I was allowed to drive the horses. When I wanted them to turn to the right or left, I would call out Gee or Haw. They knew what to do and they would turn without me having to even tug on the reins.

Grandpa chewed tobacco, but never in the house. There was a tool shed alongside the barn with the door always standing open. Just inside the door was an exposed two-by-four-foot beam, and that was where his tin of chewing tobacco was always available. As Grandpa would be going to the barn, he would reach inside the door, grab a pinch of tobacco, and tuck it inside his mouth.

Marjorie was a cousin about five years older than I was, and she was a lot more daring than me. She came to play at Grandpa's farm one summer day and she got the idea that we should mix sand into Grandpa's chewing tobacco tin. It is the only time that I can remember Grandpa being really upset, and Marjorie was sent home in a hurry!

Many of my memories of the farm revolve around food and holidays. Chocolate pie was one of my favorites, so Grandma made chocolate pie just for me. One day she asked me to bring the pie to her and on the way, it fell upside down onto the kitchen floor. As I looked at the mess that I had made, I started to cry. When Grandma saw, she went and got two spoons and said, "That pie was made for you, and you and I are going to have it." With that, she invited me to sit down on the floor beside her, and she and I ate pie. My tears soon turned to laughter.

We spent many Thanksgiving Days at Grandma's house. She would always cook the turkey with a goose. She would say, "The turkey is too dry, the goose is too greasy. You have to cook them together to get it all just right."

I enjoyed watching Grandpa milk the cows, and so did the cats, for the same reason. He would squirt milk from the cow directly into the cats' mouths and likewise into mine! The cats and I would have more milk on our faces than in our mouths, but it tasted so good!

Another thing that tasted good was Grandpa's apple cider. He made it himself as he always let it age just long enough to give it a little tang. My mother was sure that he was making alcoholics out of us, but he assured her that what he gave us was just enough to improve our digestion.

As a city boy, when I visited my grandparents in the country there was one place that I viewed with a certain fascination and yet a little apprehension. It was a building located between the toolshed and the garage. It was about one hundred yards behind the house, and it was known as the outhouse. As you entered this little building, there were two seats straight ahead. Or rather, I should say, two holes straight ahead. These were at adult height. There were two more smaller holes to the side at child height. A Sears & Roebuck catalogue was in a basket fastened to the wall. I quickly learned that to make toilet paper you needed to tear out a page and then crinkle it up into a ball. After straightening it out it became fairly soft.

During the day, the light came from a hole in the shape of a crescent moon cut into the door. At night, the light was from a lantern that Grandma would light. At first I wasn't sure that I wanted to go out all by myself at night. There was also a chamber pot under every bed. However, I soon learned that if you used the pot at night, then in the morning you had to empty it and wash it out. That was enough incentive to get me to the outhouse just before bedtime.

When I was in seventh grade my father was transferred to a church in Beloit, Wisconsin. My two older sisters were off to college and my youngest sister was getting her high school education at a boarding school. Paying for all of this education required more than my father's pastor's salary, so my mother decided to put her nursing skills to work. She took three or four nursing-home-type patients into our home, and hired one girl who lived in with us and was a great help to my mother. I helped as well. With my dad now in Beloit, I felt that I had to be the man of the house. I ran many errands. If I couldn't run them by bicycle, I would take the city bus, and in those days you could ride all over town for six cents. I remember that the school nurse checked everyone's vision and sent a note home to my mother stating that I should be checked by an eye doctor. My mother didn't drive, and my father was in Beloit, so my mother made an appointment for me to see the eye doctor by myself, and I traveled by bus. I can remember her telling me that if the eye doctor felt that I should have glasses, that I should go ahead and order a pair. It shouldn't be the most expensive pair, but it should be a pair that would hold up during my play and would not be easily broken. I have been wearing glasses ever since then.

A brand new A & P supermarket had just opened in downtown Eau Claire, and as long as I had to take the bus to the eye doctor, my mother also gave me a grocery list and told me to shop at the A & P. Normally I would have purchased the groceries at a neighborhood grocery store that was about two blocks from our home. It was always interesting to go to that place. Groceries were piled high on shelves all the way up to the ceiling. The store was a one-man operation. If the item was high up, the man would reach up with a long stick that had grabbers on the end. He would dislodge the item with one hand and catch it with the other. I waited for the day that he would miss, but it never happened while I was shopping!

Along with getting the groceries at the A & P store, my mother also had a couple of bills for me to pay while I was downtown. For me to pay these in person meant that we would save the three-cent stamp that would otherwise be placed on an envelope for each of them.

Among the patients my mother cared for that would

come and go, there was an elderly couple from Norway. The husband had the bad habit of chewing tobacco and it was my job to go to the corner grocery store and buy it for him. However, he would always give me an extra penny or two to spend on candy. At that time, for one or two cents we could buy a "Guess What," which was a candy with a little prize. And once in a great while if it was a very warm day, he would give me an extra nickel for an ice cream cone. When school was out, my mother closed up her nursing home and we moved down to Beloit and were a family again.

I started my eighth grade in a school in Beloit, where one of my classmates, Don Winger, became the brother that I never had. We have stayed in contact all these years. We still see each other on occasion, and we still communicate by telephone and e-mail. When it was time for me to start high school, my parents decided to send me to Bethel Academy, a Seventh-Day Adventist boarding school. Don Winger was going to be at the same school and we decided to be roommates.

The most significant thing that happened during my first year in that school was the bombing of Pearl Harbor by the Japanese. I walked into the dormitory that day and noticed that several students were in the dean's office listening to the radio. I joined them. I listened in astonishment to the eyewitness accounts of what was happening in Pearl Harbor. There I was, nearly fourteen years old, and a freshman in high school, and the only thing I could think of was what this would do to my plans of becoming a doctor. I soon learned that all students would be subject to the draft, with a few exceptions. If you were studying for the ministry, you would be deferred. If you were in medical school, you would be deferred until you had completed your education, and then you would be drafted.

My mother thought that if the war continued and was still going on when I turned eighteen, that I should go to divinity school so I could be deferred. If I followed her wishes, then I would take after my father and become a pastor. I pointed out to her that I had no calling to the ministry, and I felt that she was being inconsistent with her beliefs when she told me to go into divinity school strictly to be deferred. Furthermore, the thing she had always wanted me to be was a doctor, and now all of a sudden she was trying to push me in a different direction.

As I examined the effect that the war was having on education, I realized that everything was being accelerated. You could complete medical school in three years, premedical training in two years, and high school in three years. So I started informing everyone that I planned to be in medical school by the time I turned eighteen. By being there, I would probably be deferred from the draft until after I got out. And if they did draft me then, I would be an officer.

I finished my freshman school year at age fourteen. When I started my sophomore year, I decided to take extra subjects that I would normally have taken in my junior year. I took the remainder of my junior subjects in summer school following my sophomore year, and I graduated from high school at age sixteen.

The boarding school that I attended was a Seventh-Day Adventist high school; in those days they were very strict, particularly when it came to separation of the sexes. It was coeducational and I had a girlfriend. What that meant was that there was a girl who I was allowed to invite to one or two programs during the school year. We would occasionally stop and talk in the hallways. We passed notes back and forth and sometimes had a brief opportunity to hold hands. My girlfriend was a minister's daughter, and I'm a minister's son, so we started out with something in common. Her sister also had a boyfriend, and he was much braver, and much more worldly than I was. He claimed to have figured out a way that we could sneak out of the dormitory and meet our girlfriends at a cemetery that was about a block down the road from our school. There was a farm associated with the school, and the farm boys who got up for milking the cows left the dorm at about four A.M. His plan was for us to get up and leave the dormitory at the same time that the farm boys left. He didn't have an alarm clock though, so he said I would need to go along and meet my girlfriend, too, and that I'd have to be the wake-up person for him.

The night came, and I set my clock so I'd be able to wake him. The girls agreed. Around four o'clock in the morning on a cold, damp morning, the girls managed to sneak out of their dormitory, and my alarm clock didn't go off! I don't know whether it was a conscious or unconscious decision, but I didn't wake up until the rising bell at six A.M. and everybody was up!

The girls had waited down in the cemetery until they got too cold to wait anymore. They were pretty disgusted with us at that point. They went back into the dormitory, complaining all the way about what we had done to them. They complained to many of their classmates, and it wasn't long before everybody in the dormitory knew what had happened. And it wasn't long after that when the faculty knew about our misadventure. Soon I got a call from the principal to come into his office. He sat me down and began telling me how terribly against the rules it was to sneak out of the dormitory and particularly to meet with girls in the middle of the night. "But," I answered, "I didn't do this." His retort was that since it had been my intention, that was the same as if I had done it. Then he continued by saying, "It is very obvious to me that you only had one thing on your mind." And I asked him what that might possibly be, because I really wasn't sure what he thought I had on my mind. Well, he told me in no uncertain terms. I was a senior but I was only sixteen years old, and I was very naïve. I swear to this day that the things that he told me that I had on my mind had actually never entered my mind! He went on to say that I was not setting the right example for the other students, and I'd have to resign from two of the three offices that I held. I was the Sabbath School Superintendent and I was the Student Association President, and I turned in my resignations to both of these offices. However, I had just been elected president of the senior class, and he allowed me to keep that job.

After graduation, I went immediately into summer school at Andrews University in southern Michigan, and I started the premed program. At the time it was a two-year diploma program. I had one summer and one school year until my eighteenth birthday. It looked like the war was not going to be over, so I needed to be in medical school for deferment. During the school year, I applied to the University of Illinois Medical School. When the end of the school year was approaching, as was my eighteenth birthday, I received a conditional acceptance to the class starting in August. I was missing one course, they told me, histology. I went to the histology professor, and told him all about what was happening, and he agreed that when the regular semester was finished, he would teach me histology over a two-week period because I could not add it to the work load that I was carrying at that time. But before I could take my histology class, my eighteenth birthday came, and I registered for the draft. Then I took the two-week course in histology. I presented all this information, along with my conditional acceptance, to the draft board, and they said, "Greetings! You will report for duty."

At that time I was disappointed, in part because my mother was so eager for me to stay out of the service, and in part because I had been working so hard toward getting into medical school. But as I think back on it, it was a blessing. I needed a break from school, I needed time to grow up and to mature, and I needed time to sit back and let somebody else tell me what to do. I can't think of a better place for that than the army. And that's where I went.

I was off to Fort Sheridan in Illinois. My mother was sure that something terrible was going to happen to me, but truth be told, I was looking forward to a new adventure. One of the first things I did was ask for overseas duty. I felt it would be an ideal way to see the world, but as is typical in the army, I never got the chance to leave the States!

Basic training was at Camp Crowder, Missouri, and then I was transferred to Fort Sam Houston to be turned into a Surgical Technician or, as we called it, a Bedpan Commando. We finished our basic training and were to depart by train from Neosha, Missouri, in the middle of the night for San Antonio, Texas, where Fort Sam Houston was located. There were about thirty soldiers in our group. A group leader was appointed, and held all the tickets and our orders to go to the new location. When we boarded the train, I wasn't quick enough to get a seat. The car that we boarded was almost full when we arrived. I went back down the train several cars, where I found a car that was half empty. I stretched out in the seat and promptly went to sleep.

Several hours later I was awakened by a conductor asking to see my ticket. I explained to him that I was with a group of thirty soldiers who were three or four cars up. My group leader had my tickets and my traveling papers. He informed me that the group had gotten off the train to wait for another train. The train we were on was going to San Antonio by way of Dallas. A train behind us was going by way of Forth Worth, and they had decided, because our train was so full, that they would get off and get on the other train. So here I was, with no tickets, and no travel documents, sitting in a car that I learned was reserved for black people! This was my first experience with segregation. Everyone around me was listening to the conversation between me and the conductor. The conductor finally said, "As long as you're here, stay here, and you'll get to San Antonio." A few hours went by and a new conductor wanted my ticket. I explained the whole story again and his reply was, "I know nothing about a group of soldiers that you say got off the train, and you don't ride on my train without a ticket. I don't care if you are a soldier." Those sitting around me immediately came to my defense. Then he said I could wait until the two trains were back on the same track, then I could get off and join my ticket, wherever it might be located.

Two days after getting into camp, I was called to the office. The officer who called me said, "How did you get to camp? Here's your ticket and it's never been punched or used." It turned out that when our group changed trains, they did a head count. When I wasn't there, they made no effort to find out what had happened to me. They just reported that I was AWOL!

We spent one month in training at the Brooke General Hospital and then we were given a list of eight or ten hospitals and told we could choose the one where we wanted to finish our training. All the other soldiers in my group picked the places that were the closest to their homes. There was one hospital near my home, in Battle Creek, Michigan. I had already been to Battle Creek, and I wanted to go somewhere that I hadn't been. I noticed Letterman General Hospital in San Francisco, California was on the list. I had never been to San Francisco, so that was my choice, and I spent the next two months there. Then I went back to Camp Crowder, Missouri, for a permanent assignment. When I arrived there, I was assigned to the Signal Corps briefly, and then to O'Reilly General Hospital in Springfield, Missouri. When the hospital closed, I went to Fitzsimons General Hospital in Denver, Colorado, where I stayed until my discharge at Fort Reilly, Kansas.

Did anything bad happen to me, as my mother had predicted, while I was in service? Absolutely not! There were many positive things that happened. It gave me an exposure to medicine that I feel was invaluable, and the GI bill was a real financial help as I continued with my education.

When I was discharged it was November, and too late for me to start school. There were about six weeks until the next school term was to begin. While I was in service, my middle sister was married. I had not been able to attend her wedding because I couldn't get a leave. My mother and father both wrote to my commanding officer, stating that as her only brother, I was needed for the wedding party. His only reply was, "This is not the kind of emergency that demands my attention." Only if she were dying or dead would he consider giving me a leave.

My new brother-in-law was operating the family farm. He had an old two-seater airplane called a Porterfield. He flew this plane out of a very small field across the road from his house. He called me up one day and said, "My hired man had just left me and you're going to be home six weeks before you go to school. If you'd like to come on down here to the farm and help me out, I'll find a new hired man before long. But during that time, I'd be happy to teach you

16

how to fly. We could do this in the evening after the chores are done." I jumped at the chance! I packed my bag, and I headed for Watertown, Wisconsin, where his farm was.

This farm experience was a real education for me. It was my first experience milking cows. He had a milking machine but I learned the old-fashioned way during my stay. The airplane was sitting across the road in a field that probably ran a thousand or fifteen hundred feet from north to south. It may have been one hundred feet wide. There was a fence all the way around it. At the south end of the field there was an unpaved road that was one lane, and there was a row of low trees and a power line just past the fence. My brother-in-law explained that I would learn to take off and do general flight maneuvers from his field, but when it came to landing, we would go to the local airport, which had a paved runway. It was December. The evenings were getting cool, and the days were getting short. There was not a lot of daylight left after we finished the chores.

The takeoff maneuvers were going fine. I was learning to do figure eights and stalls, and it was not going to be long before we went to Watertown to the regular airport where I would be doing my landings. During my third or fourth lesson we noticed that the wind was coming from the west, but it wasn't strong enough to affect our takeoff. I continued to practice figure eights and stalls until it started to get dark. Then my brother-in-law took over the flying and started to land from the north. Because it was getting dark, and his wind sock was not lighted, he didn't notice that the wind direction had changed and it was now coming from the north and was right on our tail. We floated along and didn't touch down until we were at least three quarters of the way down the field. The brakes on that old airplane had not been working well, and they were not up to stopping us by the end of the field. We had to take off again, and taking off downwind is difficult. We managed to get into the air, but it became obvious very quickly that we were not going to make it over the power line that we were rapidly approaching. My brother-in-law decided to fly between the fence and the power line, one wheel hit the top of the fence. We lost flying speed very quickly and plowed into the small trees, and right into the fence that went around our neighbor's field across the lane. We finally came to a rest several hundred feet into the neighbor's field. The only thing damaged outside of the plane was my brother-in-law's pride! The plane was pretty well smashed up. Under the cover of darkness, we dragged what was left of the plane, on its one functional wheel, back into his pasture. We repaired the fence, and covered all the evidence of the crash with a large tarp.

The next morning I went home. I'd had enough farming and I'd had a little too much flying. There was no insurance on the plane, but my brother-in-law was able to trade the remaining intact parts for a motorcycle. Shortly after, he decided to stop farming and go back to school on the West Coast. There, the motorcycle was stolen. I guess it just wasn't meant to be. Thirty years later I got my pilot's license and I managed to fly without any accidents for ten or fifteen years.

When I returned to Andrews University in January, I was told that the requirement for medical school was now a three-year premed diploma, and I decided to get one. In the process I met Earl Peters, who was in the same program as me. Our lives continued to run along the same track for many years, and they still do, right into our old age. Earl was a good student and he was always an inspiration to me.

I applied to Loma Linda University for medical school, and toward the end of the year I received a letter stating that because of the influx of older veterans who were attempting to get into medical school, it would be impossible to consider me until had a Bachelor of Science or Bachelor of Arts degree.

The most important thing that happened to me during that school year wasn't anything scholastic. It was meeting Rachel Magray.

Don Winger was still a close friend of mine and he, along with a cousin who I was now rooming with, would on occasion go out together, largely because my cousin was the only one with a car. My cousin, Leo Keiser, was with Rachel Magray one night that we went out. Don and I were with other young ladies and this was the first time that I noticed Rachel. Leo felt that she was very nice, and after this date he planned to date her again. A school function was coming up and he asked her to attend it with him. She refused outright! She later said that she was hoping for an invitation from another student, but that student didn't ask her. Leo felt very rejected, and I rubbed it in a little, telling him that he was losing his touch with women! He made a bet with me that I couldn't get a date with her either. I had to prove to him that I could. I did, and nine months after that, Leo and Don stood with me as we were married.

The school year started with Rachel and I living in an eighteen-foot trailer house on the edge of the campus. I managed to get a night job inspecting castings in a town about fifteen miles away from school, and I had full-time activities during the day, in addition to my schoolwork. I was running a chemistry laboratory for the pre-nursing students, and my daytime activities consisted of tutoring on the side to help the pre-nursing students get through their chemistry courses.

I majored in biology and chemistry. My idea was that if I still didn't get into medical school, then I would get a doctorate in either biology or chemistry and I would teach or become an industrial chemist. That turned out not to be necessary because the letter the next spring was one welcoming me to the Loma Linda University Medical School. Rachel went with me.

School started in September, but Rachel and I were on the road to Loma Linda in June. We picked up a new Buick from a manufacturing plant in Flint, Michigan, and I drove it out to Riverside, California for a minister. He agreed to pay for the gas if we would bring the car out to the West Coast for him. We jumped at the chance, and managed to put about 3,000 miles on it before it was in his hands. I think that much mileage was a surprise for him!

We found a small apartment with a kitchen, living room, and bedroom, all run together in one open room and a tiny bathroom separated from the bedroom. The rent was seventeen dollars and fifty cents a month!

Rachel found a job working for the hospital in Loma Linda in the Central Supply Department, and I found a job working in the hospital's Obstetrical Department. When I wasn't cleaning up after deliveries, I was making up sterile supplies. I had picked up an old bicycle to get back and forth to work. Unfortunately, it had no rear fender, and every time it would rain, my back would get all wet. I ended up walking with an umbrella when it rained a lot, and wishing that I had a car.

Finally I started looking at ads for a used car. Before long I spotted an ad that said "1936 Plymouth Coupe $55.00." At the time that coupe was thirteen years old, and I decided to buy it. I couldn't sleep the night before I was to pick up my car. It didn't matter to me that there were strange noises in the back end. The seller told me that the radio didn't work, the speedometer didn't work, and the mileage gauge didn't work. What he didn't tell me was that any time it rained, the car wouldn't start! So there I was, back to walking with an umbrella on rainy days!

I announced to my wife that I had just checked on the cost of a brand new Chevrolet, and if I ordered through a wholesale dealership back east, it would cost only 900 dollars. Of course she wanted to know where the 900 dollars was going to come from. I explained to her that when I was in the service, I had money for a savings bond deducted automatically from my pay check and sent home every month. My father put the bonds into a safety deposit box and I left it at home and didn't give it much thought. Of course she wanted to know why I hadn't told her about them sooner; here there was all this money that she could have been spending! I explained that I was just leaving it there for a rainy day and I felt the rainy day was here. I would now have a car that would help me avoid some of the rain.

Life in medical school was fun, but very busy. Our first two years were at Loma Linda, California, just about sixty miles from Los Angeles. For our last two years we moved into Los Angeles, where we made use of the Los Angeles County Hospital in our junior year and the White Memorial Hospital in our senior year. We found a place to live in the city that was a duplex with individual rooms. To us, it was huge! We rented a trailer, and pulled it behind our brand new 1950 maroon Chevrolet. There wasn't nearly enough furniture for our larger quarters, so Rachel got in the habit of going to auction sales. She still likes to do this. We gradually acquired everything that we needed.

Rachel soon had a job as a secretary for a group of doctors. Three were in obstetrics and gynecology and the fourth was an anesthesiologist. I found a job that was compatible with my schoolwork. Every evening I would go to the Downey Community Hospital, which was a hospital of fifty-five beds, and I would sleep there overnight. If emergency lab work was required or an X-ray was needed, it was my job to do it. For that they paid me eight dollars a night and my breakfast the next morning. I still remember the first X-ray that I had to take. I was in my third year of medicine, and I'd had no exposure to the process of taking X-rays. An old lady fell out of bed and needed to have a hip X-ray. The nurse who brought her down to the X-ray department was very sympathetic toward me. I can still remember her saying, "Well, if all else fails, we can always read the directions." We did it together, and the X-ray turned out pretty good.

Rachel and I were living in Boyle Heights at the time, which even in those days was a pretty rough neighborhood. One night my wife heard screams coming from across the street and she was certain someone was being murdered. Of course, I was at work. When I got home the next morning, she informed me that from then on, I was going to sleep in my own bed, and that my job was over. I had been wanting that also, and I had been really looking forward to finding an excuse to get out of that job.

One opportunity I had at the hospital during our senior year was to deliver babies. The department was set up so that ladies who already had several children would be the patients of medical students, and medical students would deliver their babies. If they were having their first baby, then the interns would do the delivery. Anyone expected to have complications or in need of Caesarian sections were delivered by the resident.

My first name is a bit unusual, and I remember a black lady who was having her eleventh baby and almost named him after me. Everything went very smoothly and quickly and she had a healthy baby. It was a boy, and she said to me, as she was lying there on the table, "It all went very well and I would like to name this baby after you. What is your name?" I said, "My name is Orris." She was very quiet for a moment, and then she said, "Oh. I think I'll call him Bartholomew." To my knowledge, no one has ever named a baby after me, and this includes my grandchildren and children.

During my senior year, I applied for a one-year rotating internship at the Los Angeles County Hospital and the Madison General Hospital in Wisconsin. Madison was closer to Rachel's parents and to my parents, and she was getting pretty lonesome for the Midwest. We could have gone to either place, but we couldn't go to both; so we ended up in Madison.

My parents decided to drive out for my graduation. We were going to load up both cars with what we could fit into them, sell off the rest of our stuff, and travel back together. We planned to take an extended trip and go up to Lake Louise in Banff, to Crater Lake in Oregon, to Glacier National Park, and back to my parents' home before I started my internship in Madison on July 1. The trunks and back seats of both cars were packed tightly, and I even added a rooftop carrier to my car. All the way up the West Coast, I worried about crossing the border into Canada and then crossing back into the United States with all the stuff that I had loaded into both cars. I wondered how we would be treated by Canadian and American authorities with all this stuff. My dad tried to reassure me that things would be okay. He pointed out that we look like honest people, and he was a minister of the gospel and would have his Bible on his front seat beside him. It was a nice trip. It was the beginning of June, but Crater Lake still had nearly eighteen feet of snow on the ground! Banff and Lake Louise were beautiful, and we saw many moose feeding along the roads.

When we reached the United States border again, the

officer asked how long I had been in Canada and where I was going from there, and then he waved me through. My father was following in his car, and we pulled over to wait for him. He was right behind me. However, several minutes went by, and he was sent to another area. Nearly an hour later, my dad finally arrived. When we were packing in Los Angeles, I had needed cardboard boxes, and went down to the tavern a couple of blocks from our place to get some. The boxes that I received from the tavern had been used to ship Canadian whiskey to the United States. The border officer saw these boxes in my dad's car, and he made my dad unload the entire car and open all the whiskey boxes that he was carrying!

On arriving in Madison, we found and rented an apartment that was three stories up. We had to haul everything we had up the steps. This included a refrigerator. There was no air conditioning, there were no windows on one side of the apartment, and the windows on the other side looked right into the windows of the next apartment. The next apartment couldn't have been more than three or four feet away. Within a week the place had become unbearable, and we were looking for a different apartment. Rachel was pregnant and the heat really bothered her. We managed to find an apartment on the ground floor and the windows actually looked out at trees and grass on both sides. There was still no air conditioning, but with cross ventilation it was livable and bearable.

It was a very busy year. Earl Peters was from Wisconsin and he decided to come back to Madison and intern with me. I remember well the first set of twins that I delivered at the Madison General Hospital. Earl and I spent one month in the obstetrical department during my rotating internship. One day a lady came in already in labor. As I checked her over, I was sure that I could hear two separate heart-

24

beats. I called her obstetrician and told him that I thought this patient was going to have twins. He assured me that I was wrong, but said he would come out and check for himself. As he listened, he said, "You know, I think you're right. You have made the diagnosis that I have missed. So you are going to deliver these babies!" Fortunately for me, everything went smoothly.

Our son Ken was born just a little more than three months after arriving at Madison and just two days before his mother's birthday.

It was a rotating internship and we could elect to have extra training in any area that we were particularly interested in. I elected to take the extra training in anesthesiology. When I was nearly finished with the internship, I took my Wisconsin State Board examination and my third part of the National Board examination. After passing both, there was going to be some delay in getting my licenses to practice.

Earl and I decided it would be good for us to start a practice together and we started looking around for a place. There was an opening in Waupun, Wisconsin, for two family doctors to take over an office. The two doctors who had been there had gone into the armed forces. We were informed that we would not be able to start practicing in Waupun until August 1 and I was finishing my internship July 1, so the hospital asked me to stay on and give anesthesia in the obstetrical department. Most of the deliveries were under analgesia, not anesthesia.

I remember one patient in particular. She was ready to have her baby. She was all draped and prepared. One of the senior obstetricians, one of the new interns and one of the nurses were gowned and gloved. They were all standing at the end of the table, and I was at the head of the table giving a little analgesia and largely coaching the patient. I instructed her that with her next contraction, she should push down hard. The contraction came, and she pushed hard—really hard! The baby went flying out of her vagina, and to the amazement of the two doctors and the nurse, the cord parted, and the baby fell into the pan on the floor. Fortunately, the baby was unhurt. Right then and there, I learned that if anything goes wrong, ever, the surgeon always blames the anesthetist!

Our licenses arrived and Earl and I went to Waupun to start our practice.

2

Starting Out

Earl and I would both be working for the State prison system in Waupun, Wisconsin in the mornings. We would be taking care of the medical needs of the inmates at a division of the prison called Central State Hospital. This is where they incarcerate the criminally insane. Our afternoons were to be occupied with our family practice in a former house that was made into a very adequate and attractive office.

Now, what is it like to be locked into your work with a group that have been declared, by the courts, as criminally insane? As I think about it, there were some good things that come to mind. You could have your hair cut for, if I recall correctly, about twenty-five cents. However, as I sat there getting my hair trimmed, I couldn't help but think about the guard in charge of the tailor shop who was killed by an inmate with a pair of scissors just before we started working there. I really wasn't worried about this happening to me. I had been appointed to the committee that determined if an inmate could now be considered sane and ready to be sent back to court to stand trial or be discharged. Very quickly, everyone seemed to know that I was the new one to impress with how completely normal they were. Another perk was that you could get your shoes shined. You would pay a couple of dollars each month and you could have your shoes shined all month long, every day if you liked. When I would arrive at work, the shoe shine man was there to meet and greet me. He would act as though nothing would please him more than shining my shoes. He suggested that I should wear a different pair every day so that I could receive his services on a daily basis.

Very quickly I realized the part of my day that was behind bars was not something that I wanted to continue to do the rest of my life, and Earl and I began to read the help wanted ads in the back of the medical magazines. It was at this point that we were contacted by V. W. Swazey from Muscatine, Iowa. He said he would love to have Earl and me join him at his clinic in Iowa. We still had time left in our contract in Waupun and Rachel was pregnant with our second child. So we decided that it probably would be best for Earl to stay on at Waupun, and for me to leave to practice medicine in Iowa. The idea was for Earl to join us in Iowa as soon as our obligations in Wisconsin were fulfilled.

About the time Rachel and I were leaving, a man came into our clinic and told Earl that he was passing through town on the way to his home in Green Bay, and he had gotten a flat tire. His car was at the edge of town, and in the process of jacking it up, he was struck in the groin with the jack handle, and he desperately needed something for pain to enable him to continue on home. Earl gave it to him, and then went home for lunch. After Earl left the clinic, the man with the pretended injury went back into the clinic and told our secretary that he knew exactly where our narcotics were and he was going to help himself! If she wanted to remain healthy, she should not interfere. When he was gone she called the police. They asked if anyone was injured and for the value of the medication that he had taken. Besides writing a report, I don't think the police did much of anything.

On arrival in Muscatine, the first thing I did was look for housing. I managed to rent a two-bedroom house that was very adequate for Rachel and me and our six-month-old son. However, when our second son arrived, the house began to feel a little small. When Rachel became pregnant again, I felt it was time to look for an empty lot and build larger quarters. As I looked around, I couldn't seem to find the right place to build. One Sunday Rachel saw an ad in the newspaper that said: "For Sale. Former Legionnaire's Park to be used as a building site 1 mi. out of town." We went out to the lot that afternoon and there were about three acres, sloping up from the road with huge bur oaks and hickory trees scattered over the entire lot. The lot had been used for pasturing sheep, and as a park. It was beautiful. It was right next door to Dr. Catalona, the only orthopedic surgeon in Muscatine. He had bought his lot at the same time that a friend of his bought the lot with the trees. His friend was then transferred out of town, and he placed the lot in the hands of a real estate agent the day before it appeared in the newspaper.

Rachel and I agreed that we wanted this lot. She said, "Make them a lower offer" and I said, "Someone else will buy it if we do." I called the real estate agent that afternoon. I told him that I would be in his office the next day with a check for the lot. He said that would be fine. The next morning, before I had a chance to get into the real estate agent's office, Dr. Catalona called me and said, "I'm very sorry, but I had planned to buy that lot and you're not going to be able to buy it." I later found out that his friend had offered it to him before putting it on the market and Dr. Catalona made a counteroffer that was about one thousand dollars lower than the friend was asking. The owner of the lot promptly called the real estate agent and offered to let him sell it. The real estate agent honored our verbal agreement, and I proceeded with my building plans.

We went to Indiana to visit my parents and while we were there, the bulldozers started digging. Then I got a call from Dr. Catalona, who said, "I still would like your lot, and I'll buy you any lot that's for sale in the city of Muscatine in exchange for your lot." I said, "Give me twenty-four hours to think about it." After talking it over with Rachel, I decided to take him up on his offer and I called him back. His response was, "I don't want your, . . . ," then several swear words, then "lot," and then he hung up. We proceeded with the digging.

Dr. Catalona's lot and my lot were part of the old Ludeman Farm. Four brothers and one sister lived there, and they farmed it together. None had ever been married. Two of the brothers and the sister had died, and that was when the two lots were sold. The two brothers continued to operate the farm but one was in poor health.

Our house was to be located the distance of about one city block from the old farmhouse. We moved in on a Monday. The following Saturday, when we were getting ready for church, I looked out the window and saw one of the Ludeman brothers running down the road. As I stood there and watched, he turned into our driveway. I opened the garage door and went out to meet him. As he rushed up to me, he said, "My brother is hurt. I think he's probably dead." With that, I got him into my car and drove up to the farmhouse. As I entered the kitchen, his brother was slumped over in a chair. He had placed a shotgun in his mouth, and the top of his skull, along with his brains, were spattered over the kitchen walls and the ceiling. I called the sheriff and the medical examiner, and I stayed until they arrived.

A year went by. I tried to be neighborly with the remaining Ludeman brother, but he pretty much kept to himself. One day he placed a note with five dollars in his mailbox, asking the letter carrier to please call the sheriff and the medical examiner and tell them that he had committed suicide. His only relative was his niece, and he had left the farm to her in his will. She put it up for sale, and Dr. Catalona bought it! There was a road in front of our house, but Dr. Catalona owned the property on the other three sides. On the side opposite his house and right next to ours, pigs were being raised.

We had a picture-perfect view from the window in our living room. The window was six feet high by about twelve feet long. It looked out at our trees. There was a bur oak tree that must have been at least eight feet wide, and it was about ten feet away from our house. The first of its limbs that went over the house was too large to put your arms around. I noticed there was some dead wood in the tree, so I called a tree specialist to come out and clean it out. I watched as he climbed up the tree. When he reached the first branch, he hollered down and said, "This you have to see!" He climbed down and went to his truck for a ladder and a flashlight. I climbed up the ladder and used the flashlight to look inside the tree, and found that it was hollow. The first limb that went out over our house was also hollow. There was only a thin shell. The tree came down; I planted flowers inside the hollow stump.

We also had a hickory tree right beside our garage, which was attached to the house. One rainy, windy day I was looking out the window and noticed that the hickory tree was swaying back and forth. Suddenly, it fell over, on top of our garage roof! That time our insurance paid for the repairs, and to have it cut up.

We moved into our new home in the fall. I managed to put in the lawn just before everything froze up. In the spring, as we looked around and surveyed our large lawn, we noticed it was almost ready to be mowed. I went out and bought my first riding lawn mower. It was a Simplicity mower that you steered with a stick, and as you pulled back on the stick, you would move forward. It made mowing almost fun! As I rode around the yard, often with my son Ken riding with me, Rachel would observe all the fun and finally she came out into the front yard and asked if she could do a little of the mowing also.

There was a telephone pole by our driveway and wire that ran down it at a forty-five degree angle. As Rachel started mowing around the edge of the lawn, I noticed that she was lined up on the wire and the pole. The closer she came to the wire, the harder she pulled on the stick and the faster she went, until the mower drove her right up the wire. And that was the last time that she used the Simplicity mower!

The practice of medicine in Muscatine, Iowa, was definitely different than in Wisconsin. Dr. Swazey's practice consisted of more welfare patients than we had been accustomed to seeing in Wisconsin. He would never turn anyone down, regardless of their ability to pay. Some of the other doctors in town limited their services to high-paying customers, so we were seeing more than our fair share of welfare patients. Dr. Swazey was very dedicated to always being available to his patients, and having the office open seven days a week. On Saturday we would take turns going down to the office from eight P.M. until ten P.M. But on Sunday morning it was a different story, and all three of us would show up for two or three hours.

My obstetrical practice was expanding. At that time we were charging seventy-five dollars for a delivery. This also included prenatal and the postnatal care, and care of the baby while it was in the hospital. Some patients couldn't even afford that. I mentioned to one of my patients the

32

day that she delivered, that she had almost had her baby on my birthday. The day she was going home was my birthday. The first thing she did when she got home was bake me a birthday cake, which her husband delivered that evening! That was my only payment, and that birthday cake could have been more than they could really afford.

Thinking of babies, I well remember that as I was cutting a baby's umbilical cord, the mother asked loudly, "Does the baby look like my husband?" Then in a more hushed tone she said, "It better look like my husband." I reassured her that she had a very fine, good-looking baby boy and I was sure it would look just like the father.

About that same time, I had just finished with my hospital rounds and I was walking out of the hospital through the lobby, when I noticed one of my pregnant patients coming into the front door on the arm of our local chiropractor. It was very obvious that she was in active labor and her delivery was imminent. I looked, but didn't see her husband. I quickly found a wheelchair and I took her up to the delivery room myself. We skipped the front desk and went straight to the delivery room. It was going to be her sixth baby and I didn't bother with any of the formalities of having her admitted. Within fifteen minutes of reaching the delivery room, we had a fine baby boy. Only then did I take time to inquire why Dr. Dobbs, the chiropractor, brought her to the hospital. She said, "He told me that when I went into labor, if I would come by his office to get an adjustment, I wouldn't need an episiotomy, and you see, I had that baby and I didn't have an episiotomy." All I could say was, "If I had only known, believe me, you would've had one!"

Not long after that, one of my patients called the office and asked to speak to me directly and, if possible, right away. She told me that she needed a house call—the sooner the better. When I asked her what her medical problem was, she said she couldn't tell me over the phone. And with the type of problem she had, she didn't want to expose everyone in my office. So around noon that day, I grabbed my medical bag and went down to a trailer park in the south end of our town. I found the right trailer and knocked on the door. I had no idea what to expect. She invited me in, closed the door behind me, and showed me a piece of tissue with a black speck on it. On careful inspection, I announced to her that the speck was probably a body louse and she began to cry. I tried to reassure her that it was treatable, that she definitely wasn't the first person to have lice, and if she didn't share clothes or combs with others, she was unlikely to pass them on to anyone else.

The area south of Muscatine was called The Island, and this is where I was asked to make a house call once for a seven- or eight-year-old girl with severe abdominal pain, nausea, and vomiting, who had no way to get to my office. When I arrived, she was lying on a couch, fully dressed. There was a kettle on the floor just in case she needed to vomit. I pulled up a chair beside her and I started to lift her dress up so that I could examine her abdomen more easily. She immediately grabbed the hem of her dress with both hands and pulled downward on it. With that, the mother grabbed her hands and said, "Don't you do that. After all, he isn't a man. He's just a doctor!"

It wasn't too long after that incident that I had the other extreme happen. The Swazey Clinic was located in downtown Muscatine, on a corner. There was a filling station in one direction and in the other direction there were several blocks of stores, most of which had two-stories, with apartments over them. The town drunk sat in a chair in front of the filling station, where he could have a fairly good look at what was happening in that area of town. I received a call from a lady who lived in one of these over-the-store apartments. She requested a house call. It was only a block away from my office so I grabbed my bag and started down the sidewalk on foot. Shortly after starting out, the town drunk came along and said that he couldn't give me any money for my services, but he could help carry my bag. I relinquished my bag to him reluctantly and he gave it back when we had reached our destination. I mounted the steps, knocked on the door, and the door swung open. Here stood my patient. She was beckoning me in, and she was stark naked! That was in the days before nudity had become common. I told her that I would wait in the hallway until she had a chance to find a robe or get back into bed.

Then there was Darlene Riviera. The Heinz Company processed its tomato products in Muscatine, and it employed many local people, and also imported workers from Puerto Rico. Darlene worked for Heinz, and in the course of her work, she met and married a young man from Puerto Rico. Darlene was big and tall. She weighed between 300 and 350 pounds. She would go on diets, and when she lost 100 pounds she would become pregnant and would put it all back on. This happened several times. She finally decided just to stay heavy so her husband wouldn't sleep with her and she would not have any more children. That way she didn't need to bother with birth control.

Darlene's husband invited his sister Anna from Puerto Rico to come and live with them. She was eager to come to the States and he knew that she could help with the children. Somewhere down the line she could probably also get a job with the Heinz company. She was tiny, I am sure not more than 110 pounds, but fiery in temperament. One day I received a request from them to make a house call. They said that Anna was upset and they would really appreciate if I could come right out and help calm her down. Upon arriving at the house, Darlene's husband was waiting for me in the yard. He showed me into the house, and in the middle of the living room floor, quietly lying on her stomach, was Anna—with Darlene, all 300 pounds of her sitting on the middle of Anna's back! I hollered at her, "Darlene! Get off that girl before you kill her!" Without saying a word she got up and moved to one side, and Anna sprang to her feet as though she had been shot from a gun. She grabbed the nearest chair and she smashed it into the television. I said to Darlene's husband, "Hold her quick while Darlene sits back down on her again!"

Iowa has doctors who perform the job of coroners, called medical examiners. Dr. Peters took on a coroner's job, and when he eventually departed from the Swazey Clinic, I inherited that job. Muscatine is on the Mississippi River and it was not uncommon to have deaths due to drowning. The sheriff called me one day to let me know that there was a body near the shore about two miles from town, and asked if I would meet him there. Upon arriving at the river, I saw a man's body pulled up on shore. The man was lying on his stomach. I could see what appeared to be a billfold in one pocket and I asked the sheriff if he would retrieve it for me. The sheriff took out a pocket knife, opened it, and very carefully cut open the pocket. Then he flipped the billfold out onto the ground, closed the knife, and threw it as far as he could into the river. His only comment was, "There's your billfold." The dead man turned out to have been missing for about three months and had probably committed suicide.

Another medical examiner case that stands out in my memory was one that I was called to see by that same sheriff. I was in church when he contacted me and he gave me directions to meet him at a farm that was about five miles from town. An older couple lived there. There were no children and no close relatives. The wife had a complete break with reality and the husband was being urged to have her placed in a mental institution. He decided that because she had never injured herself or anyone else that he was going to keep her on the farm for as long as she lived. He apparently had a heart attack when he was in bed, and he died. Now she continued to sleep with the body, wondering all the time why he was so quiet. The neighbor came by, in part because he hadn't seen any activity around the farm. When he approached the house, he could smell a horrible odor. He didn't go in, but went right home and called the police. The sheriff and I went into the house and examined the body. Then the sheriff ran from the house into the front yard and proceeded to vomit. It was very warm out, and we thought that he had probably been dead for five to seven days. The windows were open, and there were no screens. The body was covered with flies. Maggots were crawling out of his eye sockets. Then a wave of nausea began to pass over me as well, and I made a quick exit too!

I investigated the deaths that occurred anywhere in Muscatine County. If they occurred in the city, then the city police would contact me; if they occurred in the county, then they would contact the sheriff. Once the sheriff called and said that he had a farm case he wanted me to investigate. Iowa is a corn state. The corn grows tall, and this year on the farm it produced a bountiful crop, that wouldn't fit into the farmer's corn crib. The farmer built a temporary crib by placing steel posts in the ground and snow fences around the posts. While filling his temporary crib, it started to rain. He grabbed a tarp, climbed up on the pile of corn, and began to secure the tarp to the metal posts. At that moment, lightning struck the post that he was hanging onto.

The same sheriff called again for me to investigate a death that he believed occurred three to four days before. I was led into a basement where a middle-aged man had climbed up onto a chair and tied a rope around the I-beam. He had tied the other end of the rope around his neck. Then he kicked over the chair. I asked the sheriff to hold onto the body so that it wouldn't fall while I was cutting the rope. He said, "I don't think so! You just do the best you can."

Dorothy Lawe was a patient of mine. She was bookkeeper for a local firm. She had a husband and a twelve-year-old son. The family was very religious, good, and solid. There was an audit of the firm's books where she worked, and she was told by the CEO that there was a discrepancy in her books. He came to Dorothy and accused her of stealing from the firm. Later on, the auditors were able to reconcile her books and they realized that their first conclusion had been wrong. However, Dorothy came home after the confrontation, went into the basement, took a .22 caliber rifle, leaned over it, reached down, and pulled the trigger, sending a bullet through her heart.

I had a middle-aged female patient who had saved her money and invested it all in rental property. She ended up owning fourteen houses, all of which she rented out. Several of them began to need repairs, and one even needed a new roof. Muscatine has a high bridge across the Mississippi River. Instead of doing the logical thing and selling enough of her units to meet the repair needs, she drove her car to the middle of the bridge, stopped it, got out, and jumped to her death.

A little less than two years after our son Ken was born, our second son, Terry, was born. He wasn't Terry at the start. We named him Kevin at birth. My mother decided to come over to give us all a hand while Rachel was in the hospital, and for a while after Rachel had returned home. She arrived a couple of days after the delivery and announced that she knew someone by the name of Kevin and he wasn't a very nice person. And anyway, she liked the name Terry. I didn't like the name that my mother had given to me, so we probably shouldn't have listened to her, but we did, and our second son became Terry.

Just a little less than two years after that, our daughter Karyn was born and I felt she made our family complete and almost perfect.

Work was not perfect. Dr. Swazey would carry a three-by-five-inch card, and at the end of each week he would write down the number of patients that each of us saw during that week. He'd bring these figures to our attention any time he had seen more patients than we had, which was fairly often because he didn't take too much time off. When he was off for a weekend, and I would see patients that he might have had in the hospital, he would go over my orders and change as many as he could. If I ordered a sleeping pill, he would change it to a different one. Then he would go to the patient and apologize for having been gone at all!

This all came to a head when Dr. Swazey decided to go out to Seattle to the World's Fair. By this time, Dr. Peters had packed his bags and gone back to Wisconsin, planning to have a family practice in Janesville.

The secretaries who worked for us realized that there was tension building. About half of them would go to Dr. Swazey for their medical needs, and the other half would come to me. One of the secretaries was pregnant and she was seeing Dr. Swazey for her care. Her delivery date fell right in the middle of Dr. Swazey's vacation, so he suggested that she come into the hospital for an early induction of labor before he left. Our hospital had a rule that for an elective induction, patients had to have a consultation with another doctor to determine if the baby was ready to be delivered, so the induction would not cause any harm. I was making my evening rounds to my patients in the Obstetrics Department when I noticed Dr. Swazey sitting at his desk. He motioned for me to come over, and said, "I have Beverly in for an induction, and I want you to write the consult for her. There's no need for you to see her at all. She's ready for delivery." I told him to get someone else to write his consult, because I wasn't going to do it. Before the conversation ended, I told him that I was tired of the games that he was playing and I was going to leave the practice. He said, "You can't leave. Not until I have a replacement for you. You must stay at least six months more." With that I sat down, picked up a consult sheet, and wrote my resignation, effective thirty days later, and I walked out.

The next morning, as I was making my rounds, I saw Dr. Swazey. It looked as though he had probably been at the hospital all night. Again he motioned me over and said, "My induction didn't work. Beverly is still not in labor. Would you please see her and suggest what I should do at this time?" I saw her, wrote the consult, and told him that after thinking things through very carefully, I still planned to be gone in thirty days.

Now the questions, of course, were where to go, and what to do. A year before this happened I was visiting my sister in Green Bay, Wisconsin, and an ad in the local newspaper caught my eye because it was titled Medical Office Space for Rent. The space was located in De Pere, a suburb of Green Bay. My wife and I went out to De Pere, we drove around, and we noticed a tract of land that was on the banks of the Fox River, with a large "For Sale" sign on it. We got out of the car and walked down to the bank of the river, and I remember thinking I would love to have a house right here! We then visited with Vic DeCleene, who had purchased an old theater, and had divided it up into office spaces. He gave me a contract with a proposed plan about how he would make space for me in the building. On one hand, I really wanted to come to De Pere, but I had three children and a fair income right where I was. But I really wasn't happy with my present practice. I was so on the fence that I addressed and stamped two identical envelopes; one had the signed contract saying I would come, and the other said "I'm sorry, I will not be there." I had my wife take one of these and drop it into the mailbox, and then I opened the other one. It contained the signed contract. Looking back on it, I wish I had made the move right then and there.

3

Thirty Years in Wisconsin

The first thing I did after handing in my resignation was call Vic DeCleene in De Pere. I asked if he still had any office space available, and if he did, if he could make it ready for me in thirty days. He said, "I'll do my level best," and I began to pack. I was seeing patients in my own office in De Pere just six weeks later. We rented a house, and nine months after that broke ground on the banks of the Fox River for the home that we are still living in.

Shortly after I arrived in De Pere, I went to one of the local drug stores, introduced myself, and I told the pharmacist that I was planning on opening a practice just down the street. I asked him if he thought I would be successful. He said, "Are you going to dispense your own medications?" I told him that I had no intention of running my own pharmacy. He said, "Then you're going to have my support." He did indeed support me, and I was making enough to cover my expenses much sooner than I had ever planned.

I was concerned about just how big of a loan I would need to equip my office. At that time a pharmaceutical detail man came by to visit, and he pointed out that the Menominee Indians lived only thirty to forty miles away, and they had just closed a government-run hospital, and everything was for sale. My electrocardiogram, my blood pressure cuffs, my scales, and much, much more all came from there for pennies on the dollar. Rachel had agreed to work as my secretary until I could afford to hire someone else. Our daughter Karyn was five years old and I arranged for my sister to look after her while Rachel worked. Just three weeks later, I placed an ad for help and I hired Janice Bourgie. It was the first time that Janice had done anything in medicine and we learned how to do it together.

Our X-ray machine had a large weight at one end so that it could be tipped upright for fluoroscopic examinations. The patient's head would be on the opposite end of the table from the weight. There was a lever next to the floor that you stepped on, which made this all happen. I had a man with a dislocated shoulder who needed to be X-rayed. Janice took the man back to our X-ray room, and placed him on the table the wrong way, with his head at the same end as the counterbalance weight. Then she stepped on the lever that allowed the weighted end of the table to fall to the floor. I heard a very loud, "Holy Cow," ring throughout the building. I rushed back, and my patient had slid headfirst onto the floor as the table assumed the upright position. He had no visible injuries. We finally got his shoulder X-rayed and cared for him without further difficulties.

When we moved to De Pere, I was driving a two-year-old Chevrolet. When it appeared that we were going to be financially successful, I decided to go out and look for a new car. I finally decided on a Pontiac Lemans. I picked it up right out of the showroom on a Tuesday. The gas gauge showed that there wasn't much gas in the tank, so on Friday, as I was driving from the hospital on the west side of Green Bay to the two hospitals on the east side, I stopped at a filling station and filled my tank. There was a drawbridge right after the filling station, and the part of the bridge that could be raised was constructed of a lattice work of steel, which formed a bump. It was the morning rush hour. When I hit that bump, there was a BANG with a tremendous clatter. The car continued to run, so I continued on across the bridge. I went to a place where I could safely stop, and the car that had been behind me also stopped. We both got out, and the other driver said, "You have a problem." We saw that the gas tank had fallen off my car! The tank was connected only by the gas line, and I had dragged it across the metal bridge deck. I'm sure sparks were flying. The driver asked how he could help me, and I asked for a ride to the Pontiac garage. I immediately asked for my Chevrolet back, but the garage workers said it was already sold. They fastened the tank back onto the car, and claimed the only thing that was holding it in place had been the undercoating.

A couple of weeks later a horrible noise developed in the transmission. Back to the garage I went. This time they found a screwdriver that somebody had left in the transmission housing when it was being manufactured!

Two or three more weeks went by. I was coming home from church with my family when the car suddenly stopped and would not start again. The garage workers found that there was sand in the carburetor. They claimed that someone had put sand into my gas tank and from there it had gotten into the carburetor.

My wife had been driving a Mercury station wagon. I took her car in for servicing and decided to wait for it. As I was waiting, I walked around the showroom. I was looking at a 1964 four-door Lincoln Continental convertible, with a beautiful light blue color. The salesman approached me and asked me if I thought the car was new or used. I said, "It sure looks new to me." He went on to say that it had five thousand miles on it and had belonged to Victor McCormick, probably one of the richest men in Green Bay.

I liked the looks of that car, and I told the salesman so! I told him I had a practically new Pontiac Lemans at home that I'd be willing to trade in for this Lincoln if the price was right. He volunteered to come to my house, look at my car, and give me an evaluation. That evening he showed up in the Lincoln Continental convertible and I made the trade. I *think* he made it back to the garage without anything happening!

After all the trouble I'd had with the Pontiac, I decided to call Mr. McCormick and find out about this car that I'd bought. He lived only about a block from me. His housekeeper answered the phone. She told me that Victor had bought the car for her. Victor bought her a brand new car every year, and she would always tell her doctor when she traded it in and he would go down and buy her old car. She went on to say that her doctor was planning on buying the Lincoln so I could not have it. I told her that I already had it and it was mine!

We were in the process of selling our home in Muscatine and I decided to drive down in my new Lincoln. On our way back, we were approaching Rockford, Illinois, and it started to rain hard. Somebody stopped short, and I was fourth in a five-car pileup. The car that hit the back of mine was carrying a canoe on a cartop carrier. The front end of the canoe came right down through the ragtop and into our back seat. As if to add insult to injury, the police gave everyone a ticket—the first man for stopping, the rest of us for driving too fast for the weather conditions.

When the children were small, we had several dogs. We felt caring for pets would help them to become more responsible. There was a miniature collie that died while we were on vacation and I felt it should be replaced. As I thought back on my childhood and remembered the Boston bull terrier that I had loved so much, I decided to

45

get one for my children. One of the places we looked was the dog pound, and lo and behold, they had one, and all it cost us was the charge for the shots the pound had administered. It was male, and definitely had a mind of its own. It was not the sweet, lovable companion from my childhood. That dog had been female, and which I believe accounted for the difference.

When we moved to De Pere, the dog went with us. We fenced in our backyard and hoped that would keep Dutch, the name the children had given him, at home. Soon after we moved into our new house, a neighbor who was building about a block away called to tell us that the driveway he poured yesterday was now covered with dog tracks, and he thought they were probably from our dog. Not too long after that a second neighbor called to tell us that she had some pork chops on her back porch and had looked out just in time to see our dog running off with them. We tried tying him up but he would make such pitiful sounds that we just couldn't do it. Then we tried keeping him in the house, letting him out only briefly into the fenced-in backyard during the evening. The basement was at ground level and opened out to the backyard. Dutch would let out a little bark when he wanted to go out, or come in, and one of the children would go down and open the door for him. This seemed to be working. One night Terry let him out, and fifteen to twenty minutes later went down and let him in. Suddenly there was an odor of skunk in the house, and Terry admitted that as he was letting Dutch in, he noticed the smell. We had heard that a bath in tomato juice is helpful in getting rid of that odor. Dutch smelled better after the bath, but it was a week before we let any company into the house.

Winter came, and one night I went down to let the dog out. It was cold outside, and when I opened the door he turned and ran into the boys' bedroom and under the bed. I followed him and reached under the bed to grab him, and he bit me—not hard, but enough to let me know he wasn't going anywhere. We were finishing our basement at that time and I was telling one of the workmen all about my trials with Dutch. He said, "I have been admiring that dog ever since I have been here. If you're going to get rid of him, give him to me." We did, and one week later Dutch was back. He said, "I just can't get along with him." I was telling the women at the office about Dutch, and my secretary Dottie said, "I have a brother who lives about thirty miles from here who would love to have your dog." I said, "Fine, you may give it to him." She did, and as I recall, it was about two to three weeks later when Dottie came to work and said, "My sister-in-law laid down an ultimatum to my brother. She told him 'get rid of that dog or I am out of here.'" Dottie picked up the dog and was bringing him back to me when she stopped for gas. There was someone getting gas at the next pump who said, "My, what a beautiful dog." Dottie said, "Would you like to have him?" They said yes—end of dog story.

My obstetrical practice took off quickly. When I was at the peak of my deliveries, I was averaging about three per week for a total of over three thousand babies over the years. Delivering babies was fun. It was the one thing you did in medicine where people really got something for their money! However, it was bad for my sleep. It was a little bit like flying. We used to always say flying consists of hours of boredom with moments of sheer terror. Most deliveries were ordinary and very routine. Somewhere along the line it was decided that the significant other should be in the delivery room to help with the bonding. One of the first fathers who came into the delivery room to be with his wife during one of my deliveries took one look at the activity and passed out, striking his head against the tile wall as he went down! We had to stop everything and examine the concussion that he had sustained. There was another time when a delivery was approaching and I went out to the waiting room to invite the significant other in. There were two men sitting there. When I said that only one could come into the delivery area, they began to argue. If only one could come in, who should it be? I learned later that she ended up marrying the one who was with her at the time of the delivery.

Bellin Hospital is a teaching hospital and there was always lots of activity going on there during the deliveries, including one particular delivery. The husband was at the head of the table, and there were several nurses, including a student nurse to care for the baby, as well as other nurses performing all of the other activities that go along with delivery. I was almost finished making a complicated repair when the mother lifted her head up and announced loudly, "Now, you have been looking at my bottom for almost thirty minutes and I think it's about time that I see yours!" Suddenly, there was dead silence in the delivery room. Everybody looked at me, and I must confess, I was speechless.

I built a brand new office building in 1970 right across the street from St. Norbert's College. I had a large number of students who came into the office because of its convenient location. There was one young lady, a student at St. Norbert's, who called in saying that she had severe pains in her stomach. She wanted to come right away to see me. After a brief examination, it was obvious that she had a full term pregnancy in her abdomen and was in active labor! When I gave her my diagnosis, she responded, "That is absolutely impossible because I am technically a virgin." Now that was the first time for me that I had heard this phrase and I asked her what she meant by a technical virgin. When she explained the term to me, I explained the process of getting pregnant to her. Then I asked her what she was studying in school and she said, "Oh, I'm a biology major."

Rita came and joined Dottie in my office, and not long after that, Becky joined us. Rita stayed for twenty-four years. She handled the front desk very efficiently. Becky was my nursing assistant and she stayed for twenty-three years. Then Jan Nolan joined us, and was in charge of sending out the bills and doing some of the insurance work. She has been working with me for about thirty-five years. Each of the women had her own specialty but they were capable of doing each other's work, which made for a very harmonious office. Other women came and went, but these three were the ones who helped make my office a pleasant and efficient place.

I had come to De Pere to practice medicine in 1962, and Jan moved into the city of De Pere with her husband, Jim, at about the same time. At the time I was doing pre-employment physicals for all the teachers in the West De Pere School District. Jim had been hired by the school district as a coach and a driver's education teacher, and my first introduction to their family was doing Jim's physical. Then they brought their boys in to see me. They had two sons at the time. I saw Jim as a private patient around 1972. Shortly after that, he told me that his wife, Jan, was looking for a part-time job. I thought that Becky and Rita were being overworked, so I hired Jan.

If anyone was an office manager in my little office, it was Rita! For twenty-three years she not only looked after the business interests of the office, but was capable of doing any of the other jobs that might need to be done.

Rita became pregnant, and several weeks before her due date, I received a call that she was in labor and was go-

49

ing to St. Vincent's Hospital. Just then a call came in from Bellin Hospital saying I had a patient who was nine months pregnant and bleeding. She belonged to the Jehovah's Witness Church, and had instructed me repeatedly that under no circumstances would she tolerate receiving any blood or blood products. None of these things were to be given to her, ever! Shortly after I arrived at St. Vincent's hospital to check on Rita, I got a call from St. Mary's Hospital, which is all the way across town, telling me that I had a patient who was crossing the road and was hit by a car, which broke both of his legs. Well, I called for an obstetrical consult on my Jehovah's Witness patient and Dr. Tyler agreed to go over to see her, as I made a dash for St. Mary's Hospital. There I found a very sick man. He appeared to have had a fat emboli that had gone to his lungs. I managed to get in contact with an orthopedic specialist and then I dashed back to Bellin Hospital, where we delivered the baby of our Jehovah's Witness patient by Caesarian section. We stopped the bleeding. It turned out that she had a placenta previa, which is when the placenta lies in front of the opening of the uterus and a Caesarian section is the best treatment. After making the delivery I dashed back to St. Vincent's just in time for Rita's delivery. It turned out to be a tiny baby boy, right around five pounds as I recall. I felt like I could use a long vacation after that night was over!

In 1974, Jim was having symptoms that indicated that he should have a chest X-ray. The X-ray revealed a mediastinal tumor. This was biopsied, and it was found to be cancer. The surgeon felt that it had probably originated somewhere else in his body and spread from the other location to his mediastinum. The surgeon told Jim that he was unlikely to live more than six months, and was given thirty radiation treatments. Three years later, Jim began to have gallbladder problems. X-rays showed gallstones, and he was back to the surgeon to have his gallbladder removed. During his surgery, doctors noticed widespread metastic lesions and it was determined that the tumor had originated in his mediastinum and was a malignancy involving his thymus. Again, the surgeon told Jim that he had less than six months to live. Six and a half years later, Jim passed away—nine and a half years after the original biopsy. During all that time, Jim had been preparing for his funeral. This was a learning experience for me. We as doctors should <u>always</u> be optimistic, no matter how gloomy the future may look. Through the years I have repeatedly seen situations that seemed impossible, miraculously turn out for the better. God does work miracles!

The local Holiday Inn asked me if they could send transients to me who might be in need of medical care and I agreed to let them. They called me one morning shortly after, saying, "We have a guest who won't leave his room. Would you please come and see him?" When I arrived, one of the maids took me back to a ground floor room. She took out her key, opened the door, and then very quickly stepped away. The shades were pulled down, and the light was off. I stepped into the room and saw a man in bed with the sheet pulled over his head. I went up to him, introduced myself, and asked if I could be of help. All I got was a few grunts and groans. Then I pulled the sheet off his face and started all over again with my introduction. This time he responded with, "I am dead. Please leave me alone or just call someone to come and bury me." I said, "If I am going to have you buried, I have to know who you are, and where you live." He pointed toward a billfold that was on his bedside stand. He had a Rosendale address but I could not reach anyone there. There were also some addresses in Milwaukee.

As I called around, I learned that his home was in

Rosendale, that he was divorced, and that he had a brother who lived in Milwaukee. He had left Rosendale the morning before with the intention of traveling to Milwaukee, and no one knew how he had ended up in Green Bay. I left a message for his brother to call me as soon as he was found. Then I called the police and explained the situation, asking if they would pick him up and keep him in jail until I could get the next of kin involved and decide where he should be placed.

Shortly after, the police came for him. Then I received a call from his brother. I explained everything again. I suggested that he come to Green Bay, bring another person to drive his brother's car, and take him to Milwaukee for a complete psychiatric evaluation. His brother obviously didn't believe anything I said. He said, "Well, I can't come right down there. Well, maybe tomorrow and then I'll evaluate things." The next day I received another call from the brother. He was at the local jail. He said, "I don't know what to do. My brother refuses to leave the jail. He keeps saying, 'I'm dead. Just have me buried. I want to be buried right here.' " I said to him, "If he refuses to go with you, we will have to get a judge to commit him to a local psychiatric unit and the police will then take him out to our Brown County mental health facility." And that is exactly what happened. And no, he hadn't brought anyone along to drive his brother's car.

Later I received a call from St. Vincent's telling me that one of our psychiatrists had admitted a long-time patient of mine to their psychiatric floor and wanted me to come up in the morning and perform a complete physical examination on him. In the morning I proceeded to give the physical on what appeared to be a completely normal individual. In the course of the conversation I asked the patient, "Just why are you here on the psychiatric floor?"

His answer was, "Well, it's because I saw some spiders crossing the ceiling in my living room. Now my girlfriend didn't see them."

I responded, "So she brought you out here?"

And he said, "Oh, no, no! I decided to get rid of those spiders for good. I got out my gun and I proceeded to blow them way. She then quickly called the police and the police brought me out here."

I received a call on a Saturday afternoon from the father of a student who was attending the University of Wisconsin in Madison. He said that he had been asked by the university to pick up his son from his dormitory room. He was also told that school officials thought that he had been taking drugs and was having a bad trip. He asked if I would meet him at the Bellin Hospital psych unit to help him figure out what to do next. I called the hospital and alerted them that he was coming. When I interviewed him, he denied taking any drugs. Then I asked him why the university thought that he was having a bad trip. He said, "No, I am not on drugs, but I really am having a bad trip because the devil keeps appearing at my dormitory window." I asked him to describe the devil, and he said, "It's a very old lady." Then I asked him how he knew that she was the devil. His answer was, "Because she tells me to jump out the window and my dormitory room is on the second floor." We admitted him to the hospital and the psychiatrist treated him for schizophrenia. He improved. After about two weeks the doctors said he could spend a weekend at home. His mother came to pick him up and he asked if he could drive. On the way home, he steered the car toward a bridge abutment. His mother grabbed the wheel and averted a crash. The devil was still telling him what to do.

Hallucinations associated with schizophrenia are frequently auditory and it seems like they are always telling the individual to do harm. I had a patient who was the wife of a farmer outside of Wrightstown. She had two children, a boy of twelve and a girl of fourteen. She came in telling me that the radio would keep playing and she couldn't turn it off. Of course, I asked, "Was it music that it was playing or was somebody talking?" and she said, "The music I can turn off. But the talking, that just keeps on and on." The next question of course was, "What do the voices say?" She replied, "Always that I'm a bad person, I should do away with myself." We started her out on psych medications and she did very well—so well that after about six months without voices, when she could no longer afford her medications, she said that she probably didn't need them anymore and stopped taking them all. Within two weeks the voices started again. She went out to the barn and hung herself. Her twelve-year-old son found her.

I had two patients who were elderly sisters that lived together on the east side of De Pere. One had never married. When the other sister's husband died, she invited her sister to come live with her. They used an old-fashioned washing machine, one that had an attached wringer. The wringer consisted of two rollers that turned, pulling the clothes in and wringing out excessive moisture. One sister was doing the wash and putting the wet clothes into the wringer, when her fingertips got caught between the rollers. Instinctively, she pulled them out, and the skin was pulled right off one finger. Neither sister drove, so they called a cab and came to my office. I looked at the denuded finger and asked, "Where is the skin?" and the woman said, "I have no idea!" We left the injured woman at the office. I took a sterile bottle with a little saline and the healthy sister in my car and we went to their home. I went down into the dark basement, and still between the rollers was the missing skin! I reattached it and it became a successful skin graft.

In a solo family practice, it is the calls you receive at night when trying to sleep that are the most disturbing. These calls are usually from the emergency rooms or the obstetrical departments of one of our three hospitals. However, some are from individuals who are too fearful or worried to wait until morning.

My phone rang at three A.M. It was my answering service. My secretary said that she had a very distraught lady on the phone and asked if I would speak with her. It was a young lady who had been a patient of mine for several years. She started the conversation with, "I have to know if I am pregnant and I have to know right now." My question was, "Why right now?" She went on to explain that her boyfriend was in service and he was leaving for a one-year period overseas the very next afternoon. Their condom had broken, and if she was pregnant, she wanted to be married before he left. I told her that she was asking the impossible but to call me in the morning and we would talk more about it.

Having been raised by a father who was a pastor, I realized that a pastor's income, while adequate, certainly didn't allow many luxuries. I made it my policy not to charge the clergy for their medical care, no matter what faith or denomination they represented. As a result, I had many priests, nuns, and ministers of all denominations come to me. The nuns were the only group with calluses on their knees from the time they spent in prayer. However, on one occasion a nun came in and with no sign of embarrassment, explained that she had a recurrent problem with vaginal discharge. She dealt with her problem by removing the discharge with a plastic measuring spoon. In the process, the spoon had broken off its handle. She didn't want me to deal with the discharge, only to remove the spoon. This was accomplished with a few words of admonishment. "I don't mind how you deal with your discharge, just so you use something that is unbreakable."

Mr. Robert VanStratten worked for the McMonagle Lumber Yard in De Pere. They had recently purchased a used forklift, and for some reason that no one seemed to know, the safety bars over the driver had been removed from the machine. The plywood was stored in an open shed, and Mr. VanStratten was instructed to move a bundle of the plywood down from a place that was high up in the shed. The bundle consisted of at least fifty to seventy-five sheets that were four by eight feet wide. He needed to raise the forks almost to the top. He was able to pick the bundle up and move backward with it. But as he was backing up, the rear wheels hit a hole and the whole bundle tipped over, falling down on Bob's head. He was dazed but conscious.

Two of the workmen from the lumberyard came dashing into my office. They said, "We have had an accident at the lumberyard and we have the man out here in our car, but we can't get him to come into your office. Would you mind coming outside and checking him in the car?" I ran out. There was a two-door car and Bob was propped up in one corner of the back seat. It appeared to me that he had a broken neck. I said to the men, "You have gotten him this far, drive right on to the emergency room. I'll call them and tell them to be waiting for you to help remove him from your car when you get there."

Mr. VanStratten became paralyzed. He had a complete transection of his spinal cord at the C-6, C-7 level. He learned to live with his paralysis and lived for many years. He even drove a specially equipped van. Along the way he developed the largest pre-sacral ulcer I have ever seen. It went right down to the bone. He had no voluntary movement in his legs, but he did have involuntary spasms, which he hated. I sent him to see a plastic surgeon about his ulcer and he was scheduled for surgery. I assisted the plastic surgeon when the day came. I asked him, "Where are you going to get the necessary tissue to repair this defect?" He said, "I plan to cut his left leg off above the knee and fillet out the bone, and I'll use the remaining tissue for a large tissue graft." He did, and it worked as a cushion for Bob to sit on. Bob received the largest settlement on record at that time in Brown County. He deserved every penny of it!

A young lady was a patient of mine while she was growing up in the city of De Pere. She came into the office as an adult after I had not seen her in a number of years. She came to the office with a man who she introduced as her husband. She informed me that she now lived in Wausau, a city about 100 miles from De Pere. They were in Green Bay to see her husband's father, who was in the hospital and was not expected to live much longer. The husband said that just before leaving for Green Bay he had developed severe right flank pain. His doctor had determined that he had a small kidney stone that was stuck in his right ureter. He was given six Dilaudid tablets to control his pain and had been instructed to see his doctor as soon as he got back to Wausau. He produced the Dilaudid bottle, which was now empty. It said his doctor's name and that it had contained six tablets. He claimed he was on his way back to Wausau when the pain hit him, and he would like enough medication to relieve him on the drive home. I was skeptical of his request, but I knew his wife and her family, and I believed him. I asked him if he could pass a urine sample for me to look at. This he did promptly and it contained numerous blood cells. I gave him a prescription for six Dilaudid tablets. A half hour later the pharmacist from the drugstore in Pulaski, a town about fifteen miles away, called me. He said, "We pharmacists have a network and it has been brought to my attention that your prescription for Dilaudid was the sixth one that this man has obtained today, all from different doctors, and he has attempted to fill them all at different pharmacies. He was indeed successful most of the time." Then the pharmacist said, "What shall I do?" And I told him, "Call the police."

Mr. and Mrs. Jones[*] were loving, caring parents of three children. Anna was sixteen years old and going through a rebellious period in her life. She had a boyfriend who was older than her, had managed to introduce her to pot-smoking, and eventually got her pregnant. Mrs. Jones had no idea that Anna was pregnant.

It was a warm day and the house was not air-conditioned. As Mrs. Jones was leaving the house, she met Anna, who was carrying a pillow. She announced that she was going to sleep in the basement where it was cooler. Anna was actually in active labor, and she delivered, by herself, a stillborn infant that was approximately seven months' gestation. She was frightened but felt she couldn't confide in her parents. She called her boyfriend. He managed to sneak into the house undetected. He took the baby outside and buried it in the backyard. The next day, after a sleepless night, the boyfriend went to work. His boss noticed his anxiety and asked him what his problem was. He admitted to his boss that he had buried his girlfriend's baby. The boss promptly called the police, who went to the Jones' house and asked to speak with Anna. Anna was continuing to bleed profusely and admitted all that had happened. I was called, and I met Anna at the hospital. She

*This name has been changed.

was brought in by her father and the police. The afterbirth had remained in her uterus. When I removed it, the bleeding promptly stopped. After many years had gone by, I talked with Mrs. Jones. She said that Anna had never recovered from the episode. She had attempted suicide on one occasion, and had spent time in a mental hospital. Part of the trauma was because of the detective who had been assigned to Anna's case. He told her that his report could send her to jail. Or, the whole matter could be dropped if she would have sex with him.

He was eventually forced to retire from the police force for inappropriate activities. But the statute of limitations for the prosecution of his rape of Anna had ended.

During this period my children were growing up. All were good students, and by and large they were a joy to be around. It seemed that if something dangerous or daring was happening, then our son Terry was the one that was always around. For example, we received a call from a neighbor one spring day, and he said, "Look out your back window. See what your son is doing!" The ice that had been covering the river was breaking up into pieces. The pieces ranged in size from small to probably thirty feet across. Terry had taken our canoe, paddled it out to one of the smaller pieces, climbed onto it and was floating down the river. The water was still very cold and all I could think of was, what if the ice that he is sitting on breaks up? What if the canoe, which isn't tied to anything, floats away? At that time he managed to get back into the canoe and he came back to shore, where I was waiting to tell him just how embarrassed I was to have the neighbors upset about his activities?

Our house was built on the bank of the Fox River, with the basement opening out at ground level. Shortly after building the house, we put in a swimming pool, located close to the house because of the slope of the land. One warm, summer day I went out to check on the children, and there was Terry, perched up on the peak of the roof, preparing to jump into the swimming pool. There is a seven foot concrete area between the house and pool. The pool was only six feet deep where he was preparing to jump. The distance between the roof and the concrete was twenty-one feet and six inches. I said, "Terry, get off that roof! Don't you dare jump!" His reply was, "I have to jump! The roof is too hot for me to go over it with my bare feet." I hollered back up to him that if he jumped, a lot more than his feet would be burning! And he reluctantly turned and ran back to where he had placed the ladder. Not too long ago his children were swimming in the pool and I re-counted the story, and Terry confessed, "You know, Dad, I jumped off that roof many times. That was the only time you happened to catch me!"

When the children were eleven, thirteen and fifteen, we figured it was the right time to take them on a vacation to Europe. It would be three weeks on a bus with fifty other people. One of the things that stands out in memory about that trip was getting lost in the Italian Alps. Our bus driver was Belgian and our tour guide was English, and neither spoke much Italian. We were going to see where the Waldensians, a group of early Protestant Christians, had lived. The road we were directed to take started as a two-lane blacktop road, but as we proceeded up the mountain, it became only a one-lane blacktop road, and then a one-lane gravel road, and then it stopped altogether. There was a five-hundred-foot drop-off on one side and a rock cliff on the other, and there was nothing we could do but go back down the road. Everyone but the bus driver got out of the bus.

As he was slowly backing down that narrow little

road, we all walked alongside the bus. As we were descending the mountain, we came to a lane that went off toward the cliff side of the road. However, there was a Fiat car sitting right there, and there was no one around to move it. The car was locked. We tried pushing it out of the way. It wouldn't budge an inch. We all surrounded the car, picked it up, and moved it. Our bus turned around. We picked the car back up and moved it back into place. We all got back on board. Yes, we eventually found the right road.

After our children completed their educations, Rachel and I started taking one major trip each year. Our daughter became a nurse. Our oldest son went into the computer field, our middle son became a physical therapist; and my wife and I began to see more of the world. We had an opportunity to visit China and walked and ran for several hours on top of the Great Wall. One year we joined a group of OB/GYN doctors who were going to Russia to check out the practice of obstetrics and gynecology there. We had spent a few days in Moscow and we were scheduled to fly to southern Russia. We had been instructed to pack up and have our bags in the hallways by our door at seven A.M. and then to go down to breakfast. We were to be picked up after eating our breakfast and taken directly to the airport, where we would claim our bags and check in for our flight.

We had one doctor who was Austrian by birth, and practiced medicine in New York. The towels in our Moscow hotel were big, beautiful, and fluffy. They were hanging on towel warmers to keep them at the right temperature all the time. Our Austrian doctor observed the towels, and while packing up, he slipped one of them into his bag just in case they didn't have any towels in Samarkand, which was our next destination in southern Russia. He expected things wouldn't be so nice down there. When we got to the airport, he claimed his soft suitcase, which was locked.

The suitcase had been cut open and the towel was gone! Nothing else was missing, just the towel! He wanted to know what had happened. No airport employees would admit knowing anything about it. He then demanded tape to repair it. He was told that there was none available. When he asked for rope, he got the same answer. Several of us had first-aid kits. These contained Band-Aids, and we were able to make temporary repairs with them.

When we arrived in Samarkand, we went to visit a local hospital. It was one of the largest in the area and it was exclusively for the delivery and care of babies. We were to spend a little time in the delivery rooms. I was given a gown, a high baker's-type hat, a mask, and cloth boots that covered my shoes and came up to my knees. Then I went into the delivery room. It was not air-conditioned, so the windows were open, and since there were no screens, and the room was full of flies. I think they were trying to protect us from the patient's diseases, rather than the other way around.

From there we were scheduled to fly on a Sunday morning to Bukhara. Both of these places are near the Afghanistan border, and the Russians at that time were involved in a conflict with Afghanistan. Just before we retired on Saturday night, we were told that we weren't going to be flying, but we would go by train and would meet our train at midnight. When we got down to the railroad station, there were two Pullman-type cars sitting on a side track. These cars had compartments with two double-decker bunks in each. We were assigned to a compartment that was already occupied by a couple from our group. They were in bed, one above the other, and we took the opposite bunks. All this was done without one word of explanation. After a short while, the train came along and hooked onto our cars and we began to move down the track and Rachel began to cry. She was sure that they were going to haul us off to Siberia! I tried to convince her that they had no use for a bunch of American doctors in Siberia. I thought the reason we were on a train was that they didn't want us to observe their war efforts from the air.

One of our most interesting vacations was to India. The Patels lived next door to us and they were originally from Bombay. When their boys grew up the oldest decided to get married back in India. We were invited to the wedding and we decided to accept the invitation. Pravin Patel outlined what we should see in India and where we should go. Then he told us that it would take a minimum of five weeks for the trip. I had never taken off that kind of time in all the years that I'd had a solo practice. I found a young doctor who was in residency training in Milwaukee who would come up and take over my practice while I was gone. He and his wife and their small child would live in our house and he would work in my office during the five weeks that we were gone. It all worked out!

We arrived in Bombay just before Christmas and went to the Taj Mahal Hotel, which was a five-star hotel right on the waterfront. I woke up early the next morning, and while Rachel slept, I decided to take a little walk around the neighborhood. I wanted to get a taste of India—this was our first trip there. I had gone about a block and a half when I saw a man sitting on the sidewalk surrounded by several bags and two wicker baskets. He said to me, "See my snakes." I had seen snake charmers before, but never in India. So I said, "Sure." He proceeded to take the cover off one of his baskets and a cobra popped out. He had a small flute that he played for a short time, and then he covered the cobra back up. I reached into my pocket and I pulled out a five-rupee note and tried to hand it to him. He said, "No, no, no! See my mongoose." Then he took a three-foot snake out of one of his bags. He sat down on the sidewalk and out of another bag he produced a mongoose that had a string round its neck to act as a leash. The mongoose quickly went to the snake, bit it behind the head, and killed it. This was not something that I cared to witness! But I reached back into my pocket and pulled out the five-rupee note again, the one that he wouldn't take before, and once again he said, "No, no!" I tried to put the money into his hand and he placed his hand back behind himself. Then he said, "I'm a businessman and I buy my snakes. You will give me five dollars in U.S. money." I said, "No way will I pay you five dollars to see you kill one of your snakes. I do not approve of it!" And with that I turned and I started walking back toward the hotel. He reached back into his bag, pulled out another snake and began to follow after me. I'll admit, I began to walk a little faster. But he did also, and he was soon shaking that snake at the back of my head. In front of our hotel were two Sikh guards. It was obvious that they became interested in what was happening as I was approaching the hotel. The snake charmer also noticed their interest and he stuck the snake into his shirt and said, "I now take your five rupees." By then I was close enough to the guards to be brave, so I stopped and turned around and said, "You have chased me with a snake for two blocks and now you expect me to give you money! No way are you going to get any money from me!" The remainder of our trip was without incident.

The wedding was delightful. After the wedding the Patels joined us on a train trip to India's northwest desert region. We traveled on the Palace on Wheels. Prior to 1945, the Maharajas had private railroad cars that they would hook on to the end of trains to travel around the country. The Palace on Wheels car that we had was built for the Maharaja of Hyderabad in 1927. It had teak wood and silver fixtures. There were eight of us that occupied the car, plus two stewards who served us our morning meals and took care of our personal needs. For our lunches and evening meals, the train would stop and we'd walk back to a dining car to be served. The cars were lovely to look at, but we had only a large pail of water and a small cup to do our showering with. The toilet was a straight pipe that went right down to the tracks, and the wheels, when you were lying down in your bed at night, really felt as though they were square. But the trip also consisted of riding an elephant, riding camels, and seeing the beautiful desert cities, so it was truly the trip of a lifetime.

My parents were retired and living in Lake Orion, Michigan, where my sister Viola was also living. Each fall they would go to Florida and spend the winter there. They would come back sometime in the spring. In the fall of 1970 my mother called to tell me that she had a stomach ulcer. She had been having upper abdominal pain with nausea and occasional vomiting. My question to her was, "Now when you say stomach ulcers, do you mean duodenal ulcers or gastric ulcers?" She answered, "The X-ray showed it to be in the stomach." This alarmed me. Duodenal ulcers are almost never malignant. Gastric ulcers sometimes are malignant. At that time, if my patients had a gastric ulcer I would put them on a good ulcer program, take another X-ray of their stomach in three weeks, and if it showed no improvement, I would send them to a surgeon for an open biopsy. I told my mother about this and she said she didn't think surgery was necessary, but if there was no improvement, she would go to a gastroenterologist. There was no improvement, and the gastroenterologist passed a scope to biopsy the ulcer. He told my mother the biopsies were negative and it was perfectly safe for her to go to Florida for the winter. She went, but her abdominal pain continued and the vomiting was increasing. Normally my parents headed back up north to Michigan around May, but I finally convinced her to come back north in March and come directly to Green Bay instead of Michigan. When she got up to our home, we put her right into the hospital. Repeated X-rays showed the ulcer increasing in size. After surgery it proved to be a gastric carcinoma that had already spread to the regional lymph nodes. I started her on chemotherapy. She went to my sister's house, and I would go to my sister's and give her the IV medications that she needed. Not too long after her first surgery, she became jaundiced. Repeated surgeries showed that the common bile duct was obstructed with a tumor. The surgeons inserted a T-tube, which allowed the bile to drain to a pouch outside her body. This relieved the jaundice, but she grew weaker and decided to go back to her home in Lake Orion. She died August 18, 1971.

When November came, my father headed to Florida, where he had a miserable and very lonely winter. When spring came, he announced that he was never going back to Florida until he had someone to go with him. He was acquainted with a widow in town by the name of Helen Barnhardt. Fall was approaching and it would soon be time to go back to Florida. He asked if she would like to get married and go down with him. She said that she was about to leave for the West Coast to visit her daughter. He wanted to know how long she'd be gone and she said, "Oh, about two weeks." Then he told her that he would give her the two weeks to make the decision as to whether she really wanted to marry him or not. If she wasn't sure by the time she got back from California, then he would ask somebody else. However, she accepted his offer and I stood up with my father at his wedding. He married for companionship and care and she married for financial security. Money was the most important thing to her. These were not good reasons to marry. My father passed away May 4, 1980. His last years without my mother were not happy years.

The longer that I practiced, the busier that I became. This was largely due to the extra jobs that were presented to me, which I continually accepted. The first one that I took shortly after coming to De Pere was as Medical Director of the De Pere Board of Health. I continued in this position for at least twenty-five years. I also enjoyed singing in our church choir and that took one evening of practice each week. I added on the job of Medical Director of the Northeastern Wisconsin Hospice. Hospice was something that I strongly believed in and I supported it in every way that I could. The Bellin Hospital asked me to take the job as Medical Director of their Home Health Care and that meant one more weekly meeting. I was also on the staff at Brown County Mental Health Hospital. This involved mainly telephone consultations on nights and weekends. I was also Medical Director of two nursing homes. More meetings!

I felt it was getting necessary for me to cut something out and the first thing that I reluctantly gave up was delivering babies. I sent a letter to all my patients stating that I would not deliver any more babies after January first of the next year. I had arranged for the Gallaghers, who were a group of obstetricians, to come into my office on Wednesday afternoons, my afternoon off, and give prenatal care to all my patients who needed it. After January first, they would also do all my deliveries.

On January first, one of my patients, who was due on Christmas Day, decided to have a New Year's dinner with her in-laws. She lived on a farm about ten miles west of town. Her in-laws lived in Manitowoc, which is about forty miles east of town. Her mother came to look after her three children while she was in the hospital having the new baby. New Year's Day arrived and she still didn't have her baby. She and her husband loaded the children into their pickup truck, but had no room for her mother, who stayed on the farm. They started off on their way to spend the day with relatives. Just about the time they got to Green Bay, she began to have labor pains. They immediately decided to turn around, take the children back to the farm, and leave them with their grandmother. By the time they reached the farm, the pains were coming fast and hard. Grandma called the hospital and said that they were on their way and they started back to town. They had gone about half the distance to town when she announced to her husband that she felt she was going to have that baby right now! He turned into the next driveway that he saw, stopped the truck, got out, and delivered the baby right then and there. They went into the farmhouse where they had stopped and asked the people there to call me. Then they went to the hospital. I had been alerted by the hospital that she was on the way in and was in active labor. So when they arrived with their new baby, I was there, and I ended up delivering the afterbirth and tying off the cord. I told the father, "You did the hard work. This is my last baby and you did the delivery. I'm not going to charge you for this one." That was almost my last delivery. I say almost because then Becky announced that she was pregnant and I had better not give up my delivery privileges at St. Mary's Hospital because that's where she was going to go. She did, and that turned out to be the last baby that I ever delivered. When I counted them up, there were indeed over 3,000 of them. There were somewhere around thirty-five sets of twins and one set of triplets.

My job as Medical Director of the De Pere Board of Health would at times put me in strange circumstances. I can think of two different occasions when I was asked to check on homes because of unsanitary conditions.

One was the home of a large family. I believe that there were at least nine children there. No one in the family had worked for years and they were unable to find adequate housing. The city finally took on the responsibility of finding some place for them to live and they managed to rent a larger old house. Shortly after they moved in, the landlord came to the Board of Health asking us to intervene. He said, "They are living in unsanitary conditions and they are wrecking my house. Can you please help me?" I went out to check on things, and everything he had said was true. The children had knocked a hole through a wall between two rooms and they had placed a board through the hole and were using this board as a teeter totter! There were unwashed dishes, spoiling foods, unwashed clothing, and old magazines everywhere. As I was talking with the husband, he told me that he knew a place in Manitowoc where they could live, but he had no way to get there. The application for welfare in Manitowoc would definitely take time, and he didn't know what he would do for money in the meantime. The De Pere City Council unanimously agreed to continue his welfare until the Manitowoc City Council could take over, and they agreed to pay for all his moving expenses. With a collective sigh of relief, he and his family moved out of De Pere.

There was a very old, unpainted house on the west side of De Pere that had a ravine in the back. The next-door neighbors came to the Board of Health complaining of rat problems in the neighborhood. They thought that the rats originated from the old house. The City Health nurse went with me to check the home. A lady responded to our knock but she refused to let us in. When we informed her of the neighbor's complaints, she said, "We're in the process of fixing the house up and we're planning on controlling the rat infestation." Right while she was talking, several large rats scurried past us. We left and came back with the Building Inspector from the city and the police. This time we were let in to see a house with cracked windows, many leaks in the roof, piles of magazines and newspapers and evidence of rat infestation was everywhere. We had the city attorney condemn the house; it was torn down—end of rat problems!

Our oldest son, Ken, graduated from the University of Wisconsin in Madison in 1977 with a degree in Computer Science. He had been given an opportunity to work for Control Data, a firm located in Saint Paul, Minnesota. He wanted help with the moving so I borrowed a van, rented a trailer, and headed for Madison in the worst snowstorm of the year. It really was a wonder how we made it safely, both to Madison and to Minnesota. Not all of his plants made it; this was January and Ken had many plants including a prized banana tree that he had raised from a small plant. Many of them froze on the way, including the banana tree.

Our middle son, Terry, had decided to take a course in Physical Therapy and he went out to the West Coast to Loma Linda University for this course.

Our youngest child, Karyn, was going to come back to Wisconsin to use her newly acquired skills as a Psychiatric Nurse to work at St. Vincent's Hospital in Green Bay, Wisconsin.

Terry's graduation was coming up and he wanted to know if his mother and I were going to come out for it. We assured him that we were certainly planning on being there. He then asked if we had any idea what it would cost us to fly out there and stay at a hotel and eat during his graduation weekend. I tossed out a figure, and he went right on to say, "Would you please stay home and send me the money? What I would really like to do is spend time in Europe with a couple of my classmates before going to work." We went along with his request and he spent about three months seeing Europe. He ended up with eighty-nine cents in his pocket, and he said that he really didn't have much to eat the last couple of days that he was there.

Karyn was thinking that it would be nice to live at home with minimal expenses but not so nice to be right there under the watchful eye of her mother. So she decided to pack up her yellow Camaro and head for the West Coast to be close to her brother Terry, who had decided to stay out west after finishing his course in Physical Therapy. She found work in a psych hospital, but the job was at night and she didn't like working at night. A classmate of hers who was living in Florida suggested that she come to Florida where there were lots of opportunities. What her classmate didn't tell her was that she couldn't work as a nurse until she was properly registered, and that would take time. In the meantime she found work at a TGI Friday's Restaurant. There they sent her to school for a few days and then put her to work with another waitress who acted as her supervisor. What that amounted to was Karyn did the work and the other waitress took the tips!

Then the psych nurse who she had worked with in California called to tell her that he had just been hired to work for the Nevada Prison System and they needed a second nurse. She packed up her yellow Camaro and was off to Carson City, Nevada. She found working for the prison was not a job she liked. When she would go to work she was more fearful of the prison guards than she was of the prisoners. It wasn't long before she transferred out of the prison system to a job helping patients who had been released from mental hospitals. She helped them readjust to society after their hospital discharge. This work continued until she met and married a Carson City dermatologist.

Our son Ken continued with his work at Control Data. At that time they were interested in developing a super computer. They asked him to help with this development. A new company called ETA was started, specifically to develop and market the fastest computer in the world. They developed the super computer, but they couldn't market it. Times were changing, and Control Data, a company with 30,000 employees shrunk to a company with 3,000 employees, and ETA closed. The stock they had given to Ken as an incentive for him to work with them was worthless, and he was temporarily out of work. IBM was aware of what was happening to Control Data and they sent representatives to Minnesota to interview a few of the employees who had been discharged. After talking with Ken, they invited him to come to New York to look at a project that they were starting there. After he had returned to Minnesota, I phoned Ken and asked him how everything had gone. He simply said, "Not well. We couldn't get together. I have no intentions of going off to New York to sit in a little office wearing a coat and a tie, and not being paid what I'm really worth, to top it all off!" I think it was the dress code IBM had at that time that he objected to the most. Shortly after that, he was flown out to Silicon Valley and interviewed by a computer firm in Cupertino, California, and it wasn't long before they sent a truck to pick up Ken's household goods and car, and he became a West Coast resident.

When the children were small we had many pets for them: cats, dogs, rabbits, guinea pigs, even fish. As they grew up the pets grew fewer in number, until only the fish were left after the children had gone. We had a fifty-five gallon tank of tropical fish. The tank was in a closet in our basement, with an opening into the main basement room.

My wife kept saying it was time to get rid of the fish. I would say, "I look after them and what are you going to do with the hole in the wall?" She responded, "I'll hang a picture over it and it isn't fair to the fish to be alone now that we are going more." Our basement opens at ground level onto a patio. On a Sunday afternoon I noticed some bugs on the patio plants. I mixed the necessary sprays and sprayed all the plants for insects. This was the day I normally cleaned the fish tank, so when I was through with my spraying, I began to change the fish tank filter. The spray must have stayed on my hands because the next morning every one of the fish were dead. That is how my thirty years of raising fish ended. We now have a nice picture of fish hanging right there on the basement wall.

One of the trips we took at that time was to the Amazon jungle. We went to Lima, Peru, where we stayed on the ninth floor of a very modern hotel that had electronic locks that opened with a card. The Shining Path were active, and they destroyed the hotel's electrical supply. We found ourselves walking up to the ninth floor and then we needed to find a chambermaid who would have a key to get us into our room. We didn't stay there very long, but we moved on to Iquitos, which is on the Amazon River. We actually had a chance to live right out in the jungle in thatched roof huts. They were equipped with mosquito nets that came down over our beds at night. The huts were up on stilts with a veranda at one end. At sundown the lamplighter would hang a lighted lamp on the veranda and when the oil ran out, we'd better be in bed because there was no more light until morning! There was a boardwalk between the huts so we could avoid the bushmaster snakes. We were instructed to find ourselves some heavy sticks to use when we walked to protect ourselves from the snakes. We contacted two different native tribes during our stay there. I had come equipped with several flashlights and a Polaroid camera. My camera became a real hit with the natives and I used the flashlights to trade for blowguns and other items that they possessed. The blowguns were complete with darts that were tipped with poison. The natives demonstrated just how effective they could be.

We proceeded to travel down several small streams that eventually got us back on the Amazon. Suddenly, as we were slowly going along, two very modern fiberglass boats roared by. Each had two large outboard motors on the back. We were informed that these were drug runners. They were on their way to Ecuador, which brings me to our experience with drugs. We had planned to visit Machu Picchu on this trip and reserved and paid for two nights at a hotel there. This involved flying to Cuzco. Cuzco is located in the mountains. We flew from the jungle to Lima, which is at sea level. When we got off the airplane in Cuzco, we were at 12,000 feet above sea level. Then we went up to our hotel and up to the town for my wife to do some shopping. Suddenly the effects of the altitude hit her. She had nausea, vomiting, and headaches. When we arrived back at our hotel, she felt and looked miserable. The desk clerk, on observing her, said, "I'll send some coca tea, to your room. You'll feel lots better then." He did, and she did. He sent enough for me, too, so I tried it and the headache I was getting went away. Now coca tea for those who don't know, is made from the same leaves that cocaine comes from. When we were getting ready to leave Cuzco, my wife said, "I'm going to take some of that tea back to the States just so I can have something on hand in case my stomach gets upset." I assured her that the authorities would frown upon this and it really wasn't such a good idea.

We were planning to take a taxi to a small town with a market, and the next day to catch the Narrow Gauge Railroad that is the only way to get into Machu Picchu. When we arrived at the railroad terminal, we were informed that it had been disabled by the Shining Path and the only way we could go further was by walking. Now it was eighteen miles up the mountains. I asked if we could use horses but the railroad personnel said there were too many bridges. There were no roads, and the horses couldn't go over the railroad bridges. We didn't get there; we were so close and yet so far.

We had made reservations at a hotel in Machu Picchu and it took me nearly six months to get my money back. Iquitos has no roads to any other area. To leave, you have two options. One is by water and the other is to fly out. We were flying out and our flight was overbooked by eighteen people. This was on the Fawcett Airline, a local airline in Peru. Our seats had someone sitting in them and when we showed these folks our tickets with the seat number on them, they showed us their tickets with the same seat numbers.

However, they most graciously got up and gave us the seats. When it came time to depart, it was evident that the eighteen people who were overbooked had not only shown up, but they had been allowed to board the plane! The stewardess announced in three languages that we couldn't take off until all the people who were standing up in the aisles would get off the plane. The people responded by sitting down in the aisles! The stewardess made a second announcement in Spanish, Portuguese, and English. No one moved! Next, the pilot came out. He didn't speak English so I'm not sure what he said, but it was a little more forceful. No one moved! Next, the police came and they started to carry the people off, one by one. The extra people were taken away and our plane finally took off.

I was reading a medical journal and noticed an announcement for a medical meeting to be held in Rio de Janeiro, Brazil. It was in the spring, at the same time that Carnival was being held there. I've always heard that if you think Mardi Gras in New Orleans is a big party, then you should really go to Carnival in Rio, and we decided to go. Nearly four million people from around the world were reported to be at Carnival that year. Four miles of the downtown area were blocked off and bleachers were set up on both sides of the street. We obtained tickets at fifty dollars each for one night. The activities started about ten P.M. and they went until about eight o'clock the next morning. This went on every night for a week. The night we were going had finally arrived and we set off with my camera. The cab let us off at the field where the various floats and groups were assembling. There was lots of activity but there were no lights. We crossed the dark field toward the area where the bleachers were and arrived at what turned out to be an exit, not an entrance. The exit was one of those that went in one direction only, and that's out. We went up to the guard at the gate and showed him our tickets and asked where we could find our seats. He responded in Portuguese with much hand gesturing. I had no idea what he was trying to convey to us. A nearby policeman was standing and observing all that was going on and finally he came over, tapped me on the shoulder, and motioned for Rachel and me to follow him. Then he went to the exit and forcibly pulled the interlocking iron bars apart and gestured for us to go in. We did very quickly, to see thousands of seats and thousands of people, and we had no idea where our seats were located. We walked along until we found a place where there were people standing, and we stood along with them. We never did find our seats.

Rachel was sure something bad was going to happen to us and it took her about fifteen minutes until she was saying, "I have seen enough. Let's go back to the hotel." It took me about two to three hours to get to that point. Somewhere around one A.M. we went back to the exit, across the dark field to the dark street, and waited for a cab. A Volkswagen beetle stopped in front of us. The driver threw open the door to reveal that he had removed the front passenger seat to make it easy for us to get into the back seat, and he gestured for us to get in. I told him the hotel that we wanted to go to. I held up the amount of money I was willing to pay. He appeared to agree with everything and we got in. The tires squealed and we were off! He then reached under his seat and pulled out a mask which covered his entire head. He continued driving with one hand. The other hand, and his head were out the window, and he proceeded with much hollering to drive down the street. It soon became evident that he had been drinking. We'd only gone about half a mile and when I noticed that there was a solitary street light with a couple of men standing under it. He halted the cab, jumped out and joined them. We did not want to be in a cab with a drunk driver, but we also did not want to be out in the streets of Rio at one A.M., particularly with an expensive camera hanging around my neck and obviously being American tourists. The activity of stopping at a street light about every half mile continued and I finally realized that he was asking directions! He had no idea where he was going! I had been in Rio long enough to have a general idea where we were and I was able to communicate the direction that we should be heading. We made it safely back to our hotel.

There was another time that we were afraid we were not going to get back to our hotel. I decided to take a course in tropical medicine that was to be taught in English at the University of Mexico in Mexico City. When we were there, Rachel heard about a straw market she wished to visit. The hotel concierge got us a cab and told the driver where to take us, and the drivers left us at a huge market. After a couple of hours of shopping and purchasing a few baskets, we went out to the street and hailed another cab. We told the driver that we wanted to go to the Continental Hilton Hotel. The driver shrugged his shoulders and drove off. We hailed another cab. The same thing happened. The same thing happened with a third cab and I really began to wonder if we were going to get back to the hotel at all! It was obvious that with my American accent, they were not able to understand me. At that point Rachel remembered that she had a postcard to mail that had a picture of our hotel on it. I hailed yet another cab and showed the driver the card, and we were on our way back to our hotel safe and sound.

We really didn't spend all of our time vacationing. In fact, most of my time was with patients. People with many different and sometimes difficult problems were coming to me to see how I could be of help to them. One of these was Mrs. Smith.* She was a new patient. She came in with a complaint of vaginal bleeding and pain when she attempted to have intercourse. She had recently been married and felt that her problems were due to the fact that she was a virgin. She had gone to a doctor who put her into the hospital and did a D & C procedure in which the mouth of the uterus is dilated and the inside is scraped out to determine if there is any cancer or other abnormal tissue. Following this procedure she continued to have difficulty.

As I examined her, I could find no vagina. I could find no uterus. There was a patent urethra, the tube that leads from the bladder to the outside. I thought that this was the

---

*This name has been changed.

source of her bleeding. I thought that she must not have understood what her former doctor had told her. The next day I pulled her records at the hospital and behold, he described how he had dilated her cervix and had curetted her uterus and said that he was unable to determine the source of her bleeding. I explained the situation to her and offered to refer her for the plastic construction of a new vagina. She declined. I offered to talk with her husband about what was happening when they attempted to have relations, but he declined. Later when she had gallbladder surgery, it was determined that she had normal ovaries but no uterus or vagina. She was able to adopt a baby and I heard no more complaints of pain and bleeding.

Our son Terry was able to find work in southern California after he graduated from his physical therapy course. He soon had a steady girlfriend and settled down there. I received a call from him telling me that he had just been skiing up in the Lake Tahoe area near his sister's home. He had been with several other of his friends. While he was there, his temperature had gone up and he had come down with influenza-type symptoms. Terry belonged to an HMO. As soon as he arrived back home he went in to their Urgent Care Center. They told him that he had the flu and started symptomatic treatment. He finally convinced the doctors to put him in the hospital. I called and talked to his doctor. He seemed very uncertain about what was going on. We had planned to go out to southern California in about a week for a medical meeting. As I talked with Terry, he sounded confused and very sick. I decided to leave right then.

When we arrived in California we were going to stay in Terry's apartment. One of the very first things I noticed was that he had a parrot. The parrot was a gift to Terry's girlfriend. He had bought it at a local flea market. Psittacosis is a disease of birds that can be passed on to humans, and I couldn't help wondering if there could be a connection between Terry's bird and his illness. We checked the phone book and found a veterinarian's office that was not too far away. The only box I could find for the bird was a very large one. I loaded the parrot into the box and we were off to the vet's. As I sat in his office waiting room, I was completely surrounded by cats and dogs. I was the only one holding a large box on my lap with a bird in it. I couldn't help but wonder just how much this fellow knew about birds. When it was my turn to go in, I set my box down on an examining table and opened up the top. The vet reached in and felt the bird's breastbone. He immediately said, "This is a sick bird. It has no pectoral muscles. That should be the bird's most prominent chest muscle." I told him about our son's illness. He agreed the bird could have Psittacosis. He then said, "There are two ways we could go in order to find out for sure. We could draw blood from the bird and send it in to the lab and we will have a report back in about four days. Or we can sacrifice the bird and we would know tomorrow." I said, "Sacrifice the bird." He did, and the report was positive for Psittacosis. Terry was started on intravenous Tetracycline and started on his long road to recovery. I started a little Tetracycline by mouth myself in order to try to stop those bad bugs from getting to me.

At that time I was sixty-two years of age. This is an age that at one time I had felt would be a good time to retire and I began to wonder just how to go about this. My health was beginning to give me some problems. I had eaten at a Chinese restaurant on a Thursday evening and on Friday we were planning to go to a church camp for one week out in the country in small cabins. During the course of the day I developed increasing abdominal pain. I was blaming it on the restaurant where I'd had that evening meal.

Friday night I lay in bed wishing that I was back up in De Pere again. Not wanting to disturb my sleeping wife, I lay there fighting off the nausea that was coming over me in waves. Just as soon as she woke up on Saturday morning, I announced that we were going back to De Pere and she was going to drive and I'd be lying down in the back seat.

I felt every bump in the 115 miles back up to Green Bay and we went straight to the Bellin Emergency Department. I asked for Dr. Swelstad, the main surgeon who I had referred my patients to. Not only was he an excellent surgeon, but he was also a personal friend. We had played tennis together for many years. He was in surgery at that time and it took him about two more hours before he finally had a chance to see me. I had a history of diverticulosis and his feeling was that I had probably developed diverticulitis, which is when pockets in the large intestine became inflamed and may sometimes perforate. He continued on. "You have two choices and I'm going to let you make that decision. We can operate on you right now. We are dealing with an unprepared bowel so you would need a colostomy. This would be temporary," he assured me. No more than six or eight months. Or, I could have a nasogastric tube inserted and I'd be started on antibiotics to see if the perforation would seal over. I elected the second choice. Right then a colostomy didn't seem like a good idea. So the nasogastric tube went down and I started the IV antibiotics and got sicker. As they were taking me up to my room, the nurses became alarmed and called Dr. Swelstad. He increased the morphine that I was getting and everything just seemed to fade out. I was only partially aware of what went on during the next forty-eight hours. There was a CAT scan done, a barium enema given, and a trip to the operating room taken on Sunday evening.

When I finally awoke, I was in the intensive care unit and it was Monday morning. I was told that I had ruptured my appendix and peritonitis had developed. I'd had surgery, but they were unable to close my abdomen because of the infection. Things gradually improved. Finally it was time for me to go back to a general room. I still had my nasogastric tube in, I had a catheter in my bladder, and I had a central venous catheter in my vena cava to measure my pressure and to give me hyperalimentation. My abdominal incision was still draining copious amounts of purulent material and they had a heart monitor on my chest which broadcast my vital signs back to the intensive care unit.

I pleaded with my nurse, "I'm getting better. I'm out of the intensive care unit. Isn't there any of this stuff that I can get rid of?"

She said, "Well you don't need the chest monitor, but your doctor didn't order it to be taken off."

I said, "By all means, call him and get an order to have it removed!"

"We can't call for things like that. You'll just have to have it on and wait until he makes rounds tomorrow morning and we'll ask him then."

The next day came, the doctor came, and he said, "Sure. You don't need the chest monitor. It can come off." As soon as he left, I rang for my nurse.

I said to the nurse, "He agrees, the monitor comes off."

"Well, let me check." Shortly after she was back with the news that the monitor was not ordered to be removed and therefore it would have to stay!

I said, "Call him."

"I can't. It's something too minor for me to bother him

with." I thought, *this might be minor to the nurse, but it sure is major to me!* When the nurse had left the room, I carefully removed the monitor pads from my chest and laid the whole thing over on my bedside table. Of course, up in the ICU where they were monitoring the monitor, they got a straight line! Very shortly, a crash cart with all the attendants was there in my room to see if I was dead! They changed the rules after that as the result of my experience. Anyone leaving the ICU had the monitor removed unless the doctor in charge specifically wrote in his orders not to remove it.

About that time I began to develop a chronic cough. The pulmonologist said it was asthma and started me on several asthma medications. We needed to go out to my daughter's to help care for the grandchildren. She lives at an elevation of 5,500 feet just west of Carson City, Nevada. The first night that we were there, I began to have atrial fibrillation and I felt that it was probably due to all of the asthma medications that I was taking and to the elevation. The first episode only lasted for a couple of hours. I reported it to one of the cardiologists in Green Bay when I had gotten back home. He said if it happened again to call him. It happened again and after a complete workup it was decided that my fibrillation was due to idiopathic hypertrophic subarortic stenosis or IHSS. Nowadays they just call it hypertrophic myocarditis.

Next I had trouble swallowing and the gastroenterologist said that my cough was not due to asthma, but was due to gastric esophageal reflux disease. Along with all of this, I started having rectal bleeding and was told that I had ulcerative colitis. Then I discovered that my cholesterol was way too high and my PSA, or prostatic specific antigen, was also elevated. That was when I seriously began to think about retiring from everything that I was doing. I had a chance to sell my building and to sell all my equipment, and I did it. Thanksgiving Day, 1992, was my last day of work in De Pere, Wisconsin. I retired from all of my side jobs. I sent a letter to my patients asking what they wanted me to do with their charts and I locked the door. Rita and Becky had found other jobs and Jan was helping me pack up my things. Rachel had gone out to the West Coast to help our daughter with the children and I was going to follow as soon as I had finished tying up all of the loose ends.

I love to snow ski and water ski but had never had enough time for it. About the middle of December, while we were busy finishing up at the office, I noticed on TV that the Iron Mountain ski hill was opening up. That was about 100 miles north of De Pere. I was retired and didn't have to go down to that office even though I was still busy packing things. I was going to take the day off and go skiing!

The next morning I went downstairs to the closet where we kept all of our ski stuff during the summer. I pulled out my ski clothes, my skis, and a pair of yellow Nordic ski boots. I took off for Iron Mountain. After getting there I discovered that I had my wife's yellow Nordic boots. They were the same color as mine and in the dark closet I had pulled out the wrong ones. I discovered this when I was trying to put them on but failed to do so. I went to the rental shop and was informed that I had to rent skis in order to rent boots. After only two runs down the hill, my feet were killing me. The boots were too small; they put pressure on all the wrong places. I went back to the rental shop for bigger boots. The new ones were much too big! My feet would turn, but the skis would go in a different direction. I announced to everyone, and no one in particular, that this was no fun at all and I was going home! I gave my skis, boots and ski clothing to the local Goodwill store and that was the end of my skiing!

I began to make some changes in my new retirement. I lost weight, became a vegetarian, had a prostate biopsy which was negative for cancer, and had four dilatations of my esophagus. I had tubes in all places, pills of all kinds, and suppositories in both ends and I actually began to feel better!

However, the prostate continued to give me some trouble. I was getting up three or four times every night to urinate and I decided to go to one of the Green Bay urologists who had been a tennis partner of mine. I explained my symptoms to him and he said, "I think you need your prostate out. But before we do that, I need to look up into your bladder. Now we can do that today and we'll schedule your surgery for next week." He took me into a fairly large room with an examining table in the middle and a couple of chairs along one side, and I sat down in one of the chairs to wait.

Shortly after, a young lady came in. She was probably about one-third of my age. She announced, nonchalantly, "Now, take off everything from the waist down." She began to take things out of a cabinet and place them on a table. I waited for her to leave the room, or at least produce a gown or sheet. But she just continued to work. She would occasionally glance in my direction. She finally looked up and said, "Well you can leave your shoes on." I continued to wait. Then she went over to the examining table and tapped on the end of it, saying, "Put your bare heinie right here, and I mean now!" I did; no respect, no respect!

I had Dr. Swelstad come in and repair my inguinal hernia at the same time that my prostate was removed. It wasn't two procedures for the price of one, but it was one anesthetic for two procedures.

A month had passed since I had seen my last patient, and with my health improving, I became restless. There was a free clinic in Green Bay where nurses and doctors donated their time. The patients were not the very poor for whom the State provided medical care through State financial plans, but were those without insurance. They may have had jobs but they had no coverage for emergencies that would come up. For this type of patient, there was no charge. I enjoyed this and I offered to come in two days each week.

I received a phone call around then from an organization in Milwaukee. They said they heard that I was recently retired and they wondered if I was interested in doing locum tenens. I said that I wasn't interested in going out of the Green Bay area. They said, "We have openings right in Green Bay. There's an Urgent Care Center right across the street from St. Mary's Hospital. You can pick as many shifts per week as you would like. We will pay your malpractice insurance. We'll even pay you mileage to go from De Pere to your work and if you'd like to start tomorrow, you can." I didn't start the next day but about two weeks later, I did. After a month to six weeks of retirement, I found myself practicing medicine again.

One thing I hadn't been told about the job with the Urgent Care Center was that the shifts were twelve hours long. I had always insisted in my former practice that the patients make appointments, I tried to stay on time as much as possible. I encouraged patients who moved out of the De Pere area to Green Bay or some surrounding area to find new doctors, and had controlled the volume of my practice fairly well. Suddenly I was in an environment where there were no schedules, there were no appointments, and most of my patients I had never seen before. If I had a minute between sick patients, then I filled it up with truck driver's physicals, known as DOT exams, or drug screening. It wasn't long before I was sure that this was something I didn't really want to do, yet I didn't want to stay home.

It was right then and there that I remembered an article I had read in a free magazine that is sent to the doctors. The name of the magazine is "Relax." There had been an article on cruise medicine and I had clipped it out and put it into my file, telling my wife, "Now here's something for retirement." This was back in 1987. After a few months of twelve-hour shifts, I looked that article up and saw there were several addresses for the medical departments of cruise lines. Two lines had said that they hired American doctors. I wrote to both of them and eventually was accepted by both. It was about a six-month ordeal to get to the point where I received a call from Carter Hill, head of the Holland America Medical Department, saying he would like to have me join them as a physical exam doctor. At that time the Holland America Line, which we all call HAL, would place a doctor on various ships to do the annual physicals for the ships' officers. I asked if that would be all that I would be doing and he said, yes, that I wouldn't be caring for passengers. I said, "I don't think I would be interested in that." His response was that he would place my application on his assistant's desk.

He gave me her phone number and said, "If you change your mind, just phone her up and tell her."

My wife said, "You sure blew that one! You won't hear from them again."

Ten days later I received a call from the lady at HAL who actually did the assignments on the various ships. She said, "We just had a doctor that canceled out that was scheduled for the *Windstar* in the eastern Caribbean. Will you go?"

This was exactly what I wanted to do! However, we had planned a trip that was coming up that would involve driving to Branson, Missouri, to meet some friends, spending three days there listening to country music, and then driving back up to Chicago, parking our car at the airport, flying to Switzerland with a group of doctors, and touring Switzerland, France and Italy. Our expected date of return was two days after she wanted me on the ship. I told her all of this.

She came back with, "Oh, we'll just fly you from Paris when we need you." My wife was not happy with that idea. She wasn't about to have me leave her in Paris and have to come back to Chicago by herself. The HAL lady then said, "If I can get the doctor that is on board to stay two more days, then would you join the ship?" I said, "Yes."

We arrived in Chicago at eight P.M. I left Rachel on her own so she could find our car and drive up to Milwaukee, where she planned to stay with her sister, and I had an hour and a half to get to my next gate to fly to Miami, where they had reservations for me at a hotel at the airport. There I managed to get four hours of sleep, and then it was on to Barbados, where I was taken to the *Windstar*, a four-masted sailing ship with 148 passengers and ninety-two crew members.

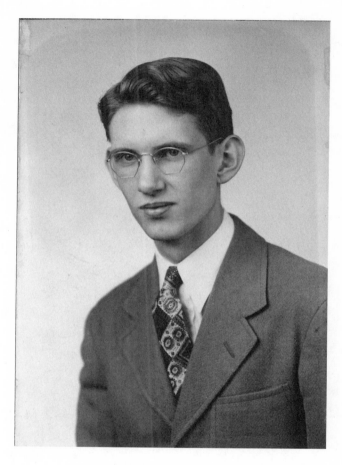

Age 16, as a senior in high school

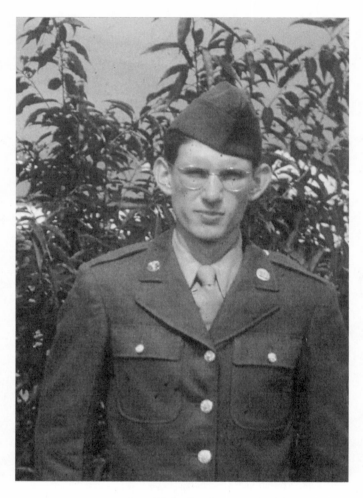

Age 18, in the Army

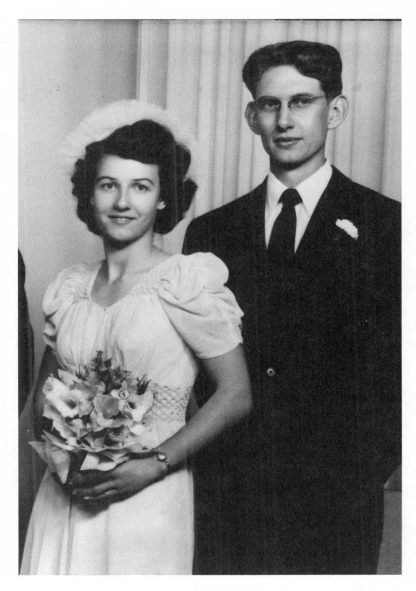

Age 21, just married

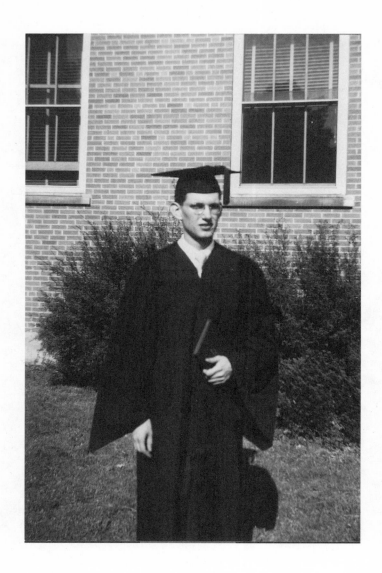

Age 22, college graduation

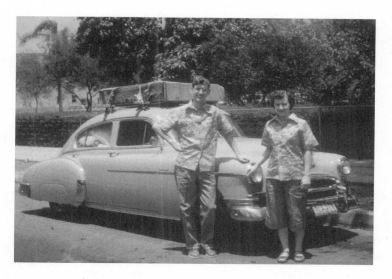

Age 26, with wife, Rachel, leaving from Los Angeles for internship in Madison, Wisconsin

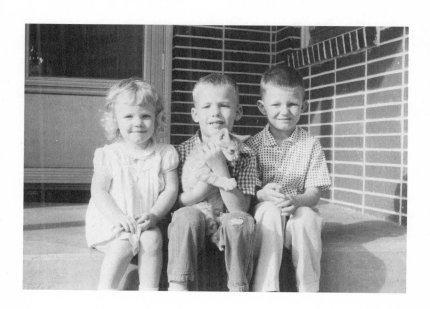

Karyn, age 2; Terry, age 4; Ken, age 6

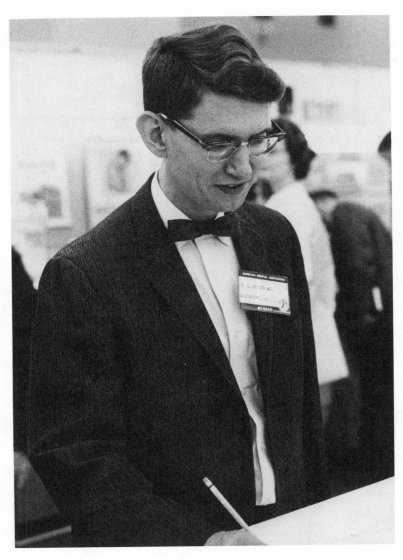

Age 34, at a medical meeting, New York City

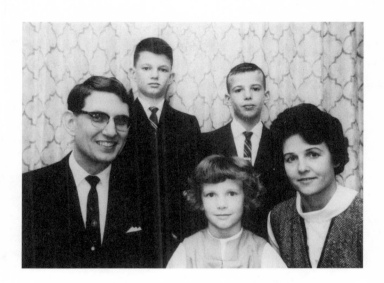

Age 38, with wife and children, ages 8, 10, and 12

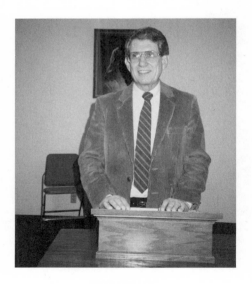

Age 48

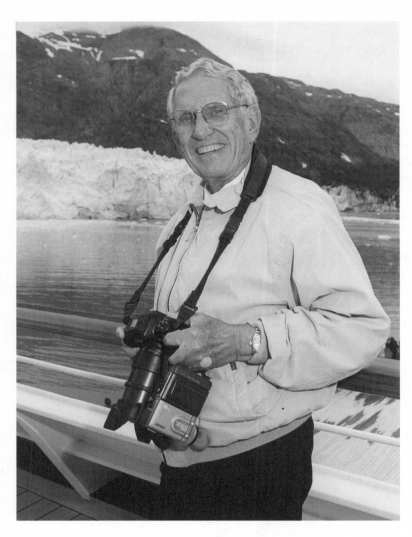

Age 74, in Alaska

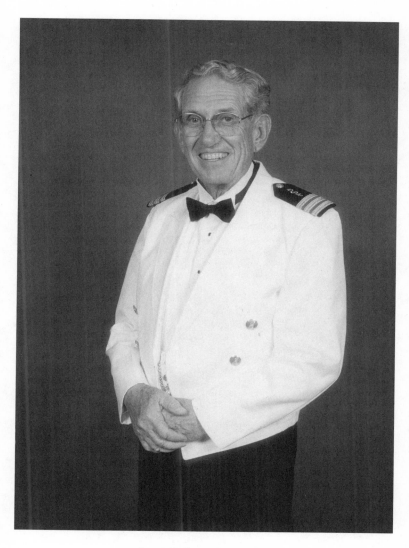

Age 74, formal uniform

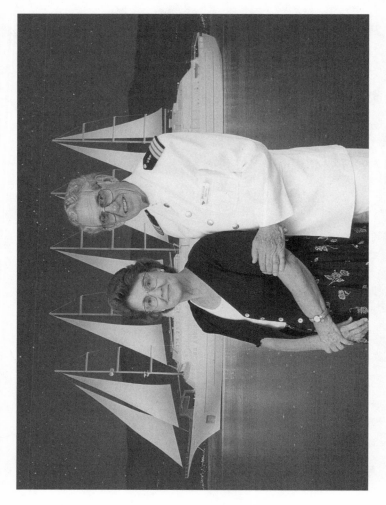

Age 75, on MS *Windsurf* with Rachel

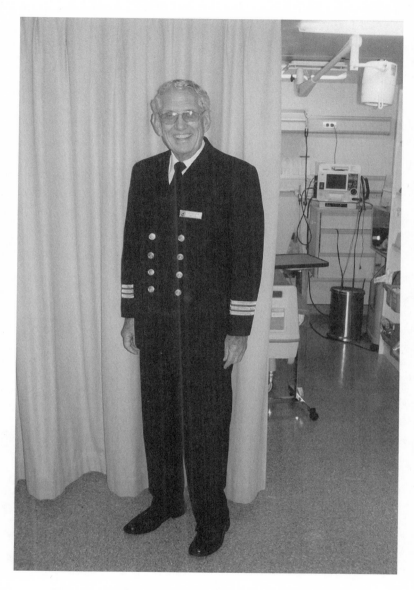

Age 76, at the ship's infirmary in cold weather uniform

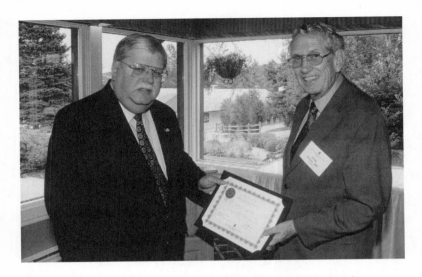

Age 76, being honored for practicing medicine for fifty years

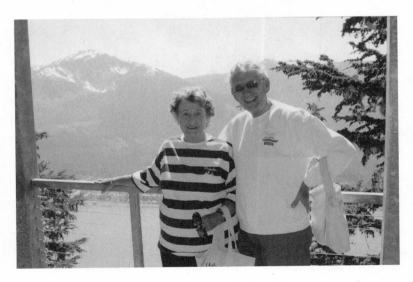

Age 77, with wife, Rachel, in Alaska

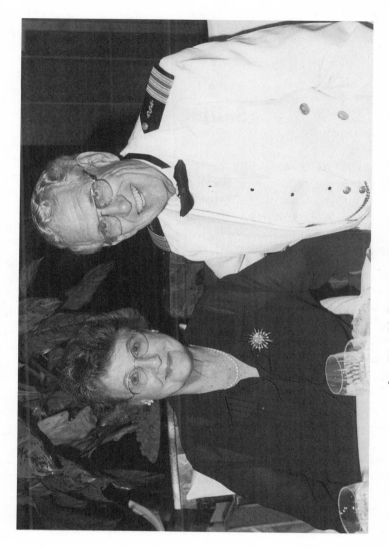

Age 77, with Rachel on MS _Prinsendam_

4

Sailing

When I got to the ship, the doctor I was replacing was gone and I was the only medical crew on board. There was no one to tell me what to do or to give me any sort of orientation. I *really* felt alone and I was going to be there for a month. It was the start of a brand new chapter in my life.

I have now been working for Holland America Line for nine years. What happened to the other cruise line that I had originally applied to? It was called the Radisson Diamond; it's now known as the Radisson of the Seven Seas. Holland America Line was the first to give me an assignment and it was obvious that I could work as much or as little as I wanted to for them. So I never did sail the Radisson Diamond ships.

My first contract consisted of four voyages that were one week each, with four different sets of passengers. One week we would go to the islands that were north of Barbados and the next week we would go to the islands south of Barbados. Some of the passengers did stay on for both the north and south voyages. I don't think I got off the ship once during that first week. There weren't many sick people, which was good. I spent the time taking inventory to see what drugs I had to use and figuring out how to order the ones that we needed or were low on. I had to learn how to make out voyage reports and the other 101 paper reports that I later found out the nurses did on the larger ships. As I learned my way around the infirmary, I would go on shore more and more, always with my radio on my belt, of course. I couldn't go beyond the radio range and that wasn't very far at times. I began to see places up close that I had never dreamed I would ever go to. After that month on the ship, I told the Urgent Care Center that I would not be back.

When I returned to De Pere, I found that Bellin Hospital had placed medical personnel in my office and I have never taken the opportunity to go back to my office since Bellin took over. This was the building that I had built in 1970.

One of the perks of my job was that after my first voyage, Rachel could join me anytime that she chose to do so. She was considered a secretary. However, she received no pay and had no duties.

My next contract was on the *Rotterdam V.* It was a stately old steamship built in 1956 and has now been replaced by the *Rotterdam VI*. There was an incident that happened shortly after I got on board. We had about 1,000 passengers and 500 crew members to look after. I had three nurses and that certainly made life easier. The passenger infirmary was separate from the crew infirmary. The nurse paged me and said, "Please come quickly to the crew infirmary. I have a bleeder here." The crew infirmary was down in the bottom of the ship. As you walked in the infirmary door, you faced the examination table. As I walked in, there was a crewman lying on the table. His pants and shorts were pushed down around his knees. There was a towel between his legs and there was blood everywhere! I quickly estimated that there must be at least a pint of blood on his clothing and the towel. I pulled on a pair of gloves and could see arterial blood pulsating from his penis. I asked the nurse for the largest needle that she had, and without the benefit of anesthesia, I began to put in a fig-ure-eight suture to control the bleeding. Only then did I take the time to ask the nurse, "What has happened?"

She said, "I haven't a clue. He doesn't speak a word of English." He was a Filipino sailor.

"Get an interpreter," I said, and she did. When the in-terpreter arrived, I asked him to find out what had happened.

He asked the sailor and then told me, "He said he had a stone in his penis."

"You mean a stone, like a rock?"

"Yes."

I asked him, "How big?" He held up his fingers to show a size of about one inch long by a half inch wide. "You are telling me that this man had someone put a stone under the skin of his penis?"

"Yes. This happened when he was seventeen years old."

"Why, under the sun, would anyone do a thing like that?"

He asked the sailor, and his response was, "To please his girlfriend."

Obviously the stone was now gone and I said, "Well, where is the stone now?"

"Oh, he took it out."

I was almost too afraid, but I asked, "How did he take it out?"

"With a double-edged razor blade!" In my fifty years of practice, that was a first and, I must say, also a last!

At that time I was sailing about six months out of the year. The majority of the physicians who were sailing the other ships were in active emergency room practices. They would come at their assigned times and usually not for more than a month at a time. I became known around the

Seattle office as one of their firemen, because I could be called on short notice.

For a number of years we had a condominium in Lake Worth, Florida, in Palm Beach County. After my retirement we started spending our winters in Florida. The home port for many of HAL's ships was at Fort Lauderdale, which was just forty-three miles from our condominium. Once I was called and told that one of the physicians was delayed in Denver due to a snowstorm and wasn't going to be able to make it on the ship the next day, and could I take his place. Then there was a doctor who showed up at the ship without his passport. I think at that time I had six hours to get ready to go down there.

The ships come into the home port at about seven A.M. They disembark their passengers, clean up, take new passengers, and sail out at about five P.M. On one occasion, the head nurse and the doctor she was sailing with didn't get along. They were both supposed to be on the next voyage. When the nurse got into Fort Lauderdale, she called Seattle and said that she would not sail again if she had to sail with that particular doctor. I think Seattle valued her more than the doctor, because they called me and asked me to take his place. It was going to be a ten-day voyage and I had a conflict, so they asked how far I could go and I said, "Well I can go as far as Saint Thomas."

And they said, "That'll give us time to find a replacement."

When we got to Saint Thomas, there was a replacement waiting for me and I flew back home.

We were beginning to see the world. In the summer of 1996 we were assigned to the *Windstar* for a month. Our home port was to be Monte Carlo and we would be doing four one-week cruises along the French and Italian Riviera. The *Windstar* held 148 passengers and ninety-two crew members. We were just beginning our fourth voyage, and at about eight A.M. I was rushing up the stairway from my cabin to the main deck when I received a page asking me to come to the bridge. As I was going up the steps to the bridge, the radio operator was coming down. He was obviously looking for me and he said, "You have an emergency call in the radio room."

We went up the steps together. I picked up the phone to hear my son-in-law's voice. He said, "The Coast Guard has just picked up a body from under the Golden Gate Bridge in San Francisco and they believe that it could be the body of your son Kenneth." Now I knew that Ken had been depressed and was seeing a psychiatrist, but I couldn't at that moment even comprehend what he was telling me.

I merely said, "I will call you back."

Then I went down to our cabin. Rachel was getting dressed and standing in the bathroom door when I told her, "They think Ken has committed suicide." We both started crying. After getting control of ourselves, I called back and learned there was a suicide note in his car. His car was parked and locked and the keys to the car were in his pants pocket and he was observed jumping from the bridge.

Now the ship cannot sail without a physician on board so the first thing I did was look over the passenger list for physicians. I discovered that there was a lady traveling with two children, and she turned out to be a Board Certified Internist. Her husband had died eight months before and this was her first vacation since his death. I explained to her what had happened and she agreed to take my place. Then I called the HAL office in Seattle and they already knew about my son and were very sympathetic. They were already making plans for Rachel and me to leave the ship

106

that day. They agreed to my appointment of the passenger to take my place.

We were anchored at the island of Elba. Later that day we took a ferry over to the mainland of Italy where we were met by a cab driver and the Port Agent, who had been sent directions for our travel from Seattle. He explained that the cab driver would take us directly to Rome. This was about 120 miles away. We were to go to a hotel where we would stay overnight. We would be catching an early flight on Alitalia Airline directly from Rome to Chicago and then on to Green Bay. The cab driver had not taken part in the conversation that we were having with the Port Agent and we presumed that he did not speak English. We were speeding along the Italian freeways at up to 120 kilometers per hour. I still don't know what that translates to in miles per hour, but it seemed pretty fast. Suddenly, after an hour or so into the trip, he spoke English. It wasn't perfect, but it wasn't bad, and he asked if we needed to use a restroom. Obviously, in a situation like ours, he hadn't known what to say either so he hadn't said anything.

I was scheduled to go out on a ship to Alaska in a little over two weeks. Everything until then went by in a blur, and when the day of the funeral arrived, I called Carter Hill, the head physician for HAL, and told him that this was the very worst day in my entire life and I didn't feel like I could go out on the Alaska voyage. He said, "No problem. If I can't find someone to take your place, I'll go myself." All my relatives encouraged me to go back to work right away. They felt that sitting around would just make my depression worse; so two days after the funeral I called Carter Hill back and said, "I can go if you still want me to."

"Fine. I have made plans to take your place myself and I'll still go. It'll be a vacation for me and I'll take along my two teenage sons."

We decided to drive out to Cupertino, and after settling Ken's affairs, we'd go to see our daughter in Carson City, Nevada, and then we would fly from there to Vancouver for our trip up to Alaska.

The funeral was indeed the worst day of my life. Sorting through Ken's things was almost as bad, but it was done. We found ourselves back at our daughter's and then back on a ship.

Our first day out of Vancouver was a sea day. On the afternoon of that sea day I was paged to see a man who was seriously threatening to jump overboard! He was a disc jockey from Philadelphia. He had a sponsor that was in the travel business and he had promoted this Alaska trip over the radio and had agreed to lead the group that was going. Seventy-nine passengers signed up to go along with him. It seemed like everything was going wrong with his trip, and he was supposed to make everything that was happening be all right. He said, "All I do is sit in a little room with a microphone and I don't know how to make it right for people." I sat down next to him and asked him to tell me all about his mother and father, who they were, what they were like, if they were still living. Then I told him about Ken. It was so fresh, so raw, that not only did I start crying, but the disc jockey started crying too. We continued to talk and it was obvious to me that he was the wrong man for this job. I asked if he would be willing to sign a contract. My part of the contract would be that I would see to it that he was sent home from our next port. I would include a letter to his boss saying that his return was at my recommendation. His part of the contract was that he would not injure himself and that he would see a psychiatrist as soon as he arrived back in Philadelphia. He readily agreed. The next morning, as he came into the infirmary to pick up his letter, he told me that he firmly believed that God had placed me on the ship to save his life.

Each year during the month of August the ship doctors would receive a "wish list." This is a list of all the voyages scheduled for the next year. Each year HAL does one world cruise—one trip all the way around the world. In 1996, when the wish list arrived, the only thing I asked for was the 1997 world cruise. It would be 103 days, starting in Los Angeles and ending in Fort Lauderdale. It was considered a reward and I wasn't sure I would get it. I had heard that there were eight physicians who had asked for it, and there were only going to be two physicians working on board. Having two physicians meant that instead of being on call twenty-four hours a day, seven days a week, I'd be on call only every other day—practically a vacation.

Carter Hill called me in early October and said he had decided to give the world voyage to two Wisconsin doctors. I was one, and the other was Jerry Salin. I had never met Jerry; however, he lived only about forty miles from me. We were going on the *Rotterdam V.* It would be the ship's last world cruise. Many of the passengers would be repeats who had done many of the world cruises already. I was looking forward to sailing one more time on the truly beautiful old steamship. It had to be sold because of the old wood paneling in the passenger cabins, and the grand staircase that couldn't be closed with fireproof doors. The day came and we set sail from Los Angeles. Dr. Salin had come on board the ship in Fort Lauderdale and was given the cabin assigned for the doctor. When I joined the ship I was to be given a passenger cabin, but the ship was full and there were no available passenger cabins. We were told that we would be sleeping in the infirmary and sharing a bathroom with the nurses until we sent someone home because of illness. After three days in the infirmary, we got a passenger cabin to move into, but it was sold at our next port, which we arrived at two days after we had moved into that cabin. So again we had to move. By that time we had sent some people off the ship because of illness, so there was another room available for us. We moved seven times before we finally had a permanent cabin assignment, which was given to us in Hong Kong! From then on, we were in the same room until we got back to Fort Lauderdale.

On our second day at sea, on the way to our first stop, which was to be Honolulu, a lady came into the infirmary. She was in a wheelchair pushed by her husband and they were accompanied by an adult daughter. She said that just since coming on board the ship she had developed trouble walking, and was now having difficulty holding up her head. She said she had a history of polio as a teenager, and I thought that she was developing post-polio syndrome. I told her that when we reached Honolulu, she should plan to go home. She stated firmly that they had planned this trip for several years, and since she was sailing with her husband and her daughter, no matter what happened to her, she was going to stay on the ship. I said, "Look. I'll tell you what I'll do. If you'll go and see a neurologist in Honolulu, and will agree to abide by his recommendations, then I will keep you on the ship providing that he will write a letter saying it is perfectly all right for you to stay here."

I never expected the woman to come back to the ship after her visit with the neurologist. But she did, and she had a letter, and it stated that the Mefloquine she was taking to prevent her from getting malaria could be causing the neurological problems that she was having. The neurologist wrote that he had called the company that makes Mefloquine and they had told him that there were five reported cases in the literature very similar to hers. We stopped her Mefloquine, but she progressively had more muscular weakness. When we were about one day away from Sydney, Australia, her breathing muscles became paralyzed and she went into respiratory arrest. The family requested that we not put her on a respirator. She quickly passed away. She was cremated in Sydney but they have a waiting period in Australia before someone can be cremated so we had to leave her body there. After her cremation, her ashes were forwarded to Perth, which is on the west coast of Australia. We picked up her ashes there and took them on around the world. The family got off in New York in April. When I was sailing in Alaska in July, I told this story to my head nurse. She told me that a week before I had arrived on the ship, the passenger's family had thrown her ashes overboard. Holland America has a zero overboard policy so they had to do this very quietly without anyone's permission or anyone seeing them.

Rachel and I were going to take a shore excursion in Bali, and when we were going to our bus I was surrounded with vendors. One had displayed a board with twenty or thirty watches on it. Most of the watches had the Rolex name on them. I noticed one in particular that looked like a very good copy of a Rolex. It had the date and the day and the stages of the moon. I pointed to it and I offered him five dollars and he of course responded, "But this is the best watch that I have. I will not take less than thirty dollars." I came up to six dollars and he came down to twenty dollars.

We continued this way until I said, "Eight dollars."

"Not a cent less than twelve dollars." As he said this, he dropped the watch I was interested in into the bag that I was carrying.

I took the watch out of my bag and gave it back to him saying, "Ten dollars and that's my last offer."

"Okay," and he dropped the watch back in my bag. I

gave him the ten dollars and I rushed to my bus that was getting ready to leave. Rachel had found a seat and I settled in beside her. I turned and asked her if she would like to see the genuine Rolex copy that I had just purchased for ten dollars. I reached into my bag and pulled a cheap child's watch that he had managed to switch with my Rolex when he dropped a watch into my bag the second time!

Later when I was in Shanghai, I was able to purchase all the Rolex copies that I wanted at the price of two for twelve dollars. I also picked up a couple of Rado watch knockoffs, which were selling for two for nine dollars. We truly live in a disposable world. I knew these watches would not run for long, and when they stopped keeping time, I would just throw them away and use a different one. Just the other day one of my Rado watches needed a new battery. I decided to replace the battery and was charged ten dollars to have it done; more than the original price for the two watches!

Before leaving on our trip, I had mentioned to our next-door neighbor, Mrs. Patel, that we were going to be stopping in India on our way around the world. She said, "Then you must stop and see my sister who lives in Bombay." We assured her that we would certainly try to get in contact with her sister. When we reached the Maldives, the islands just south of India, I went on shore, found a phone, and placed a call to Mrs. Patel's sister. The operator said, "Come back to this phone in two hours and ask for me and I will hopefully have your call completed." Two hours later she was on the line, and I told her we would be in Bombay the next day, and asked her to come aboard the ship and have lunch with us.

The next day we got a chance to give the Patels a tour of the ship and have a nice lunch in the dining room. We were staying in Bombay for two days, and when they learned this, they invited us to tour the city with them the next day.

Bright and early the next morning the Patels were waiting for us when we went on shore. The sister had married a man by the name of Patel, the same name as that of our next-door neighbors. The name Patel is a common name in India, a little like Smith or Jones here in the States. They came for us in their fairly new BMW and asked what we would like to see. I suggested that we go to a commercial laundry that I had heard about. It was a collection of 400 or 500 washtubs—nothing automatic in that laundry! When we arrived, there were very few people doing laundry because it was a holiday. It was a day when they celebrated the coming of spring and the planting of crops. They did this in part by throwing colors. Street vendors were selling brightly colored powders. These powders were mixed with an oily substance so that they could make them into balls for the purpose of throwing them at signs, posts and other objects around the town.

We arrived to see literally hundreds of open tubs used to hand wash laundry. The laundry was then placed on clothes lines or spread out on the ground to dry. I was busy taking pictures when my hostess came to me and said, "Many of the people working here today I believe to be high on alcohol or drugs, and I'm uncomfortable being here." That was enough for me and I started back to the car!

We then decided to go to the waterfront where children were playing in the water. They were dressed in ordinary clothes. No one was wearing swimming suits. It was all very colorful. My hostess and I went down the hill to take pictures at the edge of the water. Our host stayed up in the car sitting at the steering wheel and Rachel was in the back seat of the car. I had taken just two pictures when I noticed that a man was approaching from my left, with colors in a container. I turned and started to walk back up the hill. My hostess hollered at the man in his language and this seemed to anger him and he started running toward me. The engine was started and the car doors were opened. I jumped into the front seat, I slammed the door shut, our hostess jumped into the back seat, and with squealing of tires, we were off! But my window was open. He threw a ball of colors through the open window into the side of my head. I had to wash my hair three times before I could get it all out and I have *no* idea how our host managed to get the inside of his BMW cleaned up.

As we progressed around the world, we stopped at Oman, a very rich country that had just been recently opened to tourists. It was raining when we got there. The average rainfall in Oman is less than two inches per year so this was very unusual.

We then went to Yemen and tied up the ship at the same dock that later became famous when the U.S.S. *Cole* was hit by terrorists and had a hole blown in its side. We were told that we should not take pictures of the ladies that we would see walking around with only their eyes showing. This was hard for me because photography really is my hobby: it's my passion. Rumor had it that if you were caught taking pictures you shouldn't take, you might not only lose your camera, but you might even have your hand cut off!

When we came into a new port, we would frequently hire a cab driver to take us for a tour of the town. We did this in Yemen. I was busy taking pictures; I even took some of the ladies passing by. I would roll up the window of the cab so it wouldn't be obvious what I was doing. The cab driver observed me as we were going along. He suddenly stopped the cab. Two ladies were approaching on the other side of the street dressed from head to toe in black and only their eyes were showing. He motioned for me to take their picture. I leaned across Rachel to the other side of the cab, rolled down the window and raised my camera, and immediately they started waving their hands in front of their faces and they were about to turn and run when the cab driver spoke to them in their own language. Then they crossed the street and talked to the cab driver for a few moments. Then they came to our open window and asked us in perfect English where we lived and how long we were going to be in Yemen. After about five minutes of conversation, I asked if I could take a picture of my wife standing between them. They agreed. We hopped out of the cab and I took my picture. The cab driver then joined in and motioned for me to stand between the ladies and he took my picture. The pictures turned out great and I didn't lose my camera *or* or my hand!

We went on to the city of Suez, which is at the southern end of the Suez Canal. Suez is east of Cairo and we were going to take a bus into Cairo to visit the Cairo Museum and the pyramids. A short time before we arrived there, some German tourists were shot and killed in front of the Cairo Museum. We got on our bus and were ready to head to the museum when we were told that the Egyptian government was going to supply us with an armed escort and we could not leave the city of Suez until it arrived. We sat waiting for four hours before two armored cars arrived! Off we went with one car in front of our bus and one in back. We arrived at the museum to find that it was after the closing time and everything was locked up tight. However, the museum opened up just for us, after money exchanged hands!

We arrived at the pyramids just as the sun was setting and saw a laser light show in the evening. At that time the

Hale Bopp comet was right over the highest point of the largest of the pyramids. It made for an interesting evening.

Our trip was coming to an end and we were two days out of New York when we were awakened to what had to be the worst storm I have seen in the nine years that I have been sailing. I have never been seasick so I went to the Lido restaurant and ate my usual breakfast—I believe in eating a large breakfast. It was obviously an unusual day because dishes and glasses were sliding onto the floor along with the people! I went back to my cabin to pick up my camera so that I could get some pictures of all the activity and then from there I went to the crew infirmary to see any crew members that might be in need of help.

When I arrived, there was a line at the door of seasick crew members. Not all were using the bags that had been supplied for them—some were vomiting right where they stood! The area by the door has drawers that contain our supplies. These had opened and discharged much of their contents onto the floor. The crew infirmary was at the very front and the very bottom of the ship. The infirmary was making at least thirty foot excursions up and down along with a side motion.

Then I realized that I was also seasick! And I *had* to be at work! We have an anti-emetic called sea calm on board that we would give to the passengers. I figured that this would give me an opportunity to try one and I did. And believe me, it didn't calm me at all! So I took a second one, and I continued to work. We had a total of sixteen injuries. So I took a third pill. At that point the nausea improved but I became so drowsy that I found myself lying down between patients. We had one patient who had broken a hip and another that fractured her wrist. I managed to get the bones of her wrist back in alignment. I had my nurse hold the arm in position while I tried to put a cast on. All the while the boat was going up and down and back and forth. Just as I started applying the cast, my desk broke loose from where it was fastened to the wall and started crashing from one wall to the other. My nurse offered to try to stop it but I couldn't spare her from the arm so we just let the desk slide back and forth!

That evening my nausea was gone and I went down to the dining room for the evening meal. A lady sitting at the next table was thrown from her seat and hit the top of her head on the corner of our table and I had to take her down to the infirmary for stitches.

The ship had a bottle store right next to the shop that had perfume for sale. The mixture of broken perfume bottles and whiskey bottles produced a nauseating scent that could be smelled over most of the ship. My wife collects Lladro porcelain and the ship had a lovely collection, most of which had come loose from its fastenings and was lying on the floor in pieces. She offered to try to glue the lesser damaged ones back together but they assured her that the pieces would all go back to the insurance company just as they were.

Shortly after the completion of the world cruise trip, I was asked to go to Lisbon, Portugal, and go with the *Windsurf* to Barbados. The *Windsurf* is one of HAL's sailing ships. It has 312 passengers plus crew. The storm that we had gone through was too fresh in Rachel's mind for her to consider crossing the Atlantic again so soon. She decided not to go with me. We had no storms on the trip and were able to proceed under sail during four of the eight days needed to make the crossing. When we were about halfway across, I called my wife to let her know that we were under sail, that the water was smooth, and that the voyage couldn't have been better.

Just about then the captain called me up to his cabin.

He said there was a passenger, who had made this crossing four times. He had become a friend to him, and that morning two different people had come to the captain to report that the passenger was acting strangely and needed someone to evaluate him right away. The captain asked me to do this evaluation. When I knocked on the passenger's cabin door, it was answered by an elderly man dressed casually. He invited me in. I told him just exactly what the captain had asked me to do. He immediately became defensive and said all he wanted was a little help. He then gestured toward his bed and said, "You see that Negro woman and her daughter. They won't get out of my stateroom. They just stay there in bed. When I asked my room steward for help in getting them out, he rushed off to the captain and told him that I am being unreasonable." At that moment I noticed that he had a transdermal scopolamine patch in back of his left ear. I removed the patch, I washed the area in back of his ear with soap and water, and it took about twenty minutes for the lady and her child to disappear. I can't recommend the patches to control seasickness. There are too many side effects.

When I am sailing on board one of the sailing ships, I teach a class in CPR (Cardio Pulmonary Resuscitation) to all of the newly arriving crew members, regardless of what their position on board the ship is. I always start my class by telling them about an experience I was involved in on board the MS *Rotterdam*. It happened in the ocean bar. The bartender was working alone. An elderly man came in and sat down in a chair about fifteen feet away from the bartender. As he sat there, his chin dropped to his chest. His mouth partially opened and he began to drool. Then a passenger came in and sat down on one of the bar stools. He looked over toward the elderly man and he remarked to the bartender, "He doesn't look very good. Don't you think you should do something?" The bartender went over to the telephone and phoned the front desk. He then asked the front desk to page the nurse and ask her to come up to the ocean bar to check on a passenger. When the nurse answered her page, she asked if she should take a wheelchair along with her. They answered that they didn't know. The nurse wasn't at the infirmary so she went to the infirmary, then proceeded with the wheelchair to the ocean bar. She found that the elderly man was dead. We could not resuscitate him. At this point I ask each of the crew to put themselves in the place of the bartender, and we practice on a mannequin the correct CPR techniques. If only the *Rotterdam* bartender had been given similar training, the outcome might have been different.

A man named Mr. Swearingin worked at the ticket counter of Northwest Airlines in our Green Bay airport. His family were long-time patients of mine and I had delivered several children for them. Then he was transferred to the airport in Reno, Nevada. When we visited our daughter in Carson City, we would fly into and out of the Reno airport. It was always nice to see his smiling face in back of the counter, and several times, when space was available, he upgraded us to first class. When we would check in for our flight, we would always try to check in with him. We had been returning from visiting our grandchildren, and our daughter dropped us off at the Northwest gate, and Mr. Swearingin was there. He told us that they needed to bump some passengers and asked if we would like to fly out the next day. The airline would give us 500 dollars toward our next trip. They would put us up at a hotel casino, and also give us vouchers for our meals. We jumped at the chance. That evening we decided to see a show. We were seated at a booth for four people, and soon another couple sat down with us. Almost immediately the man who was sitting next to me said, "I know you." It turned out that he had been on the world cruise with me. He had come into the infirmary to have me wash out his ears. He had said that he had been digging in his ears with cotton tipped applicators and had managed to scratch his ear canal. I had told him that nothing smaller than his elbow should ever go into his ears. He claimed to have followed my advice from then on.

We were coming south from Alaska and were in the Inside Passageway, and were going through a very narrow area. It was a foggy night; the fog was so dense that the captain, the second officer, and the two Canadian pilots were all up on the bridge. It was 10:40 at night and Rachel and I had just gone to bed. Suddenly the ship tipped to the side and we were making a sharp turn! Rachel rolled out of bed onto the floor. She got up and ran into the hallway in her nightgown to try to find out what was happening. After what seemed like an eternity, but was probably less than a minute, the ship leaned and turned to the other side. I didn't know what was happening, but I knew that I was going to get dressed before leaving the room. It turned out that suddenly, out of the fog, a boat carrying a load of logs had appeared right in front of us! The turning maneuver was done in order to avoid the boat. We managed to slip past the log boat by twenty to thirty feet. There were ten injuries associated with the Big List, as it became known throughout the fleet. Most were minor. The most seriously injured person was a lady who was sitting at the last slot machine in a line of five or six machines. As the ship leaned, she slipped down the line, hitting each machine, and each machine took a little bit more of the skin from her arms and face. The near miss was reported to HAL in Seattle, and they instructed us to go up to the bridge and check everyone up there for alcohol and drugs. All were negative. When we reached Vancouver, the captain was called back to Seattle to give a report. He never returned to a HAL ship. It was only months later that we learned that the ship with the logs also had a load of dynamite on board!

We give each employee a tuberculin skin test on a yearly basis. I was on my way to Alaska with three nurses. One was only a part-time worker for HAL, and the other two were full-time employees. The part-time nurse had not worked for HAL for almost a year, and needed to have her tuberculin skin test repeated. It was found to be positive. On checking her records, her previous skin test was negative. I ordered a chest X-ray, which we were capable of taking on the ship. When I looked at her film there were two things that stood out. One was a shadow in the apex of her right lung, and the other was that she had numerous vascular clips on the same side. When I asked her about the clips, she said that she had a mastectomy for a carcinoma of the breast five years before. I immediately made arrangements to have the radiologist in Juneau, Alaska, read her X-ray. He said he believed the shadow in her lung was the result of lung metastases from her previous carcinoma. I sent her home for continued evaluation and care. About a week later we received an e-mail from her. It said, "I have good news and bad news for you. The good news is that they have found tuberculin bacilli in my sputum and the shadows in my lung are the tuberculosis and not metastatic cancer. The bad news is that you have all been exposed to tuberculosis."

We had kept the Seattle office informed by e-mail about all that was happening. The nurse with tuberculosis thought that she had acquired it in South America. She had gone on a volunteer mission trip and worked with a cook that probably had tuberculosis. One of the other nurses had the reputation of having been very friendly with a couple of the captains in the past, and it wasn't long before I saw the captain down in the infirmary, his computer is in the same network as the computer in the infirmary. He said that he had been reading our e-mails and he wanted to know all about the nurse with tuberculosis. He then confided that he had attended a crew party and had been close to one of my nurses. He wasn't sure if she was the one with tuberculosis or not. I assured him that I knew which nurse he was talking about, and to my knowledge, she was completely free of tuberculosis.

When we go to Alaska, our first stop is often Ketchican. It is known as the Gateway to Alaska. I had been on shore and was returning to the ship when I was stopped by the security officer and told that I was needed down in the infirmary. When I entered the infirmary, there was a gentleman sitting there. I estimated his age to be around sixty-five and I noted that he had a beard and was moderately overweight. He extended his hand and said, "I am Bruce Williams." I took his hand and said, "And I am Orris Keiser." I was not in uniform, so I added, "I am the physician on board." He said, "No, I mean I am THE Bruce Williams, the most listened to talk radio host in America." I must confess, I had not heard of him. Then he said, "Where do you live?" I said, "In Green Bay, Wisconsin." He said, "I have been on WNFL in Green Bay for many years. Where have you been all that time?" In spite of the awkward meeting, we became friends during the course of the voyage, and I called his cabin on the last day of the trip to see how he was doing medically, and he said, "You're going to be famous in Green Bay." I asked him why, and he went on to say that he had been broadcasting from all the Alaska ports where we had been stopping, and each time he had mentioned me. So when I returned home, I proceeded to tell my friends about Bruce Williams—and not one had ever heard him on the radio!

One of my most famous patients was Debbie Reynolds. She was going to entertain on the ship and when she was getting out of the limousine that brought her to the ship, the wind caught the door of the car and it struck her on the left side of her face. The nurses always try to have patients come down to the infirmary rather than having us go to the cabin. One reason is that it costs the passenger a lot more money when we go up to the cabin, and the other is that we are set up to handle emergencies much better in the infirmary. Debbie called down and said she would like a cabin visit to evaluate her injuries. Of course the nurse said it would be best if she would come down to the infirmary. She said, "Would you ask the doctor if he would consider coming up here?" The nurse came into my office and casually said, "Would you consider going up to Debbie Reynolds' cabin to evaluate an injury?" I said, "THE Debbie Reynolds?" and she said, "Yes." And I said, "Where's my bag?" I found her to be very charming woman with only minor injuries.

I am frequently asked, "Do you ever have any serious illnesses or is it mainly people who are seasick or sunburned?" And my reply is, we have people who die. You cannot get more serious than that.

I overheard a passenger talking to a nurse once. He said he was traveling with his mother and she had Amyotrophic Lateral Sclerosis, or Lou Gehrig's disease. This is a condition in which we see a progressive paralysis eventually leading to death. He said that she was beginning to have trouble swallowing. With that, I came out of my office and proceeded to teach him the Heimlich maneuver, which involves placing a fist over the upper abdomen, standing behind the patient, and pressing into the abdomen in a way that hopefully will dislodge any foreign object that is obstructing the airway. I demonstrated this to him and I told him to use it just in case. Two evenings later I received a call that she was choking after having eaten escargot, and the Heimlich maneuver was ineffective. It was impossible to expel the foreign body and a tracheotomy failed and she died. But she had seen Alaska before her death, something she had always dreamed of doing.

We were in Bora Bora on the *Windsong*, a sailing ship with 148 passengers, ninety-one crew members. When I'm sailing ships I always carry a radio to go ashore, and I always stay in radio range. I had decided to rent a bicycle and ride along the coast for a few miles. When I was almost back to the bicycle rental shop, my radio came to life, and someone said I was needed back on the ship. We were anchored out in the harbor and they said that a Zodiak would come for me. I quickly paid for my bicycle rental and I hurried to the dock. I could see the Zodiak coming. It seemed rather slow. Only later did I realize that the normal driver of the Zodiak was busy with the patient and the radio operator had volunteered to pick me up, and he wasn't too familiar with the operation of the Zodiak. When I arrived at the ship, I could see a passenger lying on the sports deck with active CPR taking place. He had been diving with a group of experienced divers and the dive-master. The dive they were planning was a deep dive to about one hundred feet, and when they had descended about halfway, the dive-master noted that one of the divers was going back up toward the surface. The dive-master signaled to the others to stay right there and he went back to the surface, reaching the surface at the same time as the passenger. He asked the passenger if he was all right. He assured the dive-master that he was. The dive-master then said, "Inflate your life vest and get back into the boat." He had seven divers waiting for him fifty feet down in the water, so he went back down and finished the dive. When they came back up, they found the passenger floating face down, with his life vest inflated and CPR was started, but was ineffective. I continued CPR for a while because I hate to give up. Bora Bora is French and the people there very quickly took charge and sent the body to Tahiti, where an autopsy was performed. I repeatedly tried to find out the results of the autopsy but was unable to get any information. My theory was that the passenger probably had a cardiac irregularity, which caused him to abort the dive, and when he was on the surface, went into cardiac arrest.

We were going up the east coast of South America when one of the crew members asked me for something to help him sleep. I asked him why he couldn't sleep and he said, "Well, the voices keep me awake." He said it had been almost a week now that he'd had practically no sleep.

I then asked him, "What are the voices saying to you?"

"Oh, they keep telling me to jump overboard."

That got my attention! We put him on twenty-four-hour suicide watch and I notified Seattle of the situation. They said they would send a male nurse to take him back to the Philippines for treatment at his home. Shortly after that, we received the air schedule for the escort who was to meet our ship at our next port. Our next port was a town north of Rio de Janeiro and we were to leave there at three o'clock in the afternoon. The nurse was scheduled to arrive at our ship at 1:30 P.M. When 1:30 came, we had our crewman sitting at the gangway with his suitcase packed. At 2:00 P.M. I began to think, *what if he doesn't come?* I contacted the Port Agent and asked about local psychiatric facilities. He assured me that there was one such facility and said he would come to the ship and pick up our crewman and take him there to await the arrival of the nurse. However, we would need to send a nurse along with him as far as the hospital. It was now 2:30. I called the captain and explained that the escort had not arrived. We needed to put our crewman in a local hospital temporarily and we would need to send a nurse with him to escort him to the hospital. He assured me that we were pulling up the gangway at three P.M. If the nurse was not back, she could plan to fly to the next port or get there however she could. At 2:45 a man came rushing up. He looked like he could be from South America, and I thought he was probably the Port Agent. I was preparing to tell him that this was our crewman and this was the nurse who would be going with him to the psychiatric hospital. As I began to repeat how the escort had not arrived, he said, "I *am* your escort! We had a flat tire on our way here to the ship. No phones. I had no way to let you know. I'm here for the crewman!" So with all of ten minutes to spare, they walked off and then the gangway was raised.

Saint Martin is divided right down the middle. The French own the north half and they spell the name "Saint Martin." The Dutch own the southern half and they spell the name "Sint Maarten." There is a lot of docking space on the Dutch side, so this is where the large ships go. Ships need to anchor out when they stop at the French side, so this is where the small ships go. Almost every time we would stop at Saint Martin we were in one of HAL's sailing ships and we would anchor at Marigot, the capital of the French side. There was a large open market right there and that was where Rachel would head, and I would usually climb up the hill to Fort Louis. You could always get a wonderful picture of our sailing ship from the Fort. There are lots of beaches all around the island. One in particular is world famous for its clothing-optional policy. It is called Orient Beach.

We had never gotten around to visiting any of the beaches before, and now we were finally on a larger ship that was stopping on the Dutch side. As we walked around the Philipsburg area, I commented to Rachel that we should catch a cab and take a little tour of the island. We did this frequently when we would come into a new area. Shortly after we saw several cabs in a row. We stopped at the first one and asked the driver if he would be interested in doing this for us and he said "No" but we should check with the driver of the van that was in back of him. There was a lady with two boys sitting in the back of the van. I would guess their ages to be about ten and twelve years old. We approached the driver and he said that he would be happy to take us on a tour if we wouldn't mind stopping for a few minutes at a beach. The price was agreed on and we were off.

I then turned to the driver and asked, "What beach are we going to be stopping at?"

He replied, "the Orient Beach." You could see Rachel's jaw drop.

She then looked at the two boys and turned to the lady in the back seat saying, "Do you realize that the Orient Beach is a nude beach?"

The lady nonchalantly replied, "Of course I do. I want my boys to see everything there is to see on the island." That day we did see everything there was to see on the island.

We maintained our home in De Pere even after I had closed the doors of my office and we were spending six months of the year in Florida. Theoretically we were six months in De Pere and six months in Florida, and then of course we were spending six months on board a ship, so the reality was that we spent very little time anywhere. However, De Pere will always seem like home. De Pere is a suburb of Green Bay. The highest attraction in the Green Bay area is the Green Bay Packer football team. I have been fortunate to get tickets to their home games for the last thirty-five years. These are hard to come by, and at times very valuable. My son wanted four tickets to one of the games. He asked me if I would trade a couple of the tickets I wouldn't be using for two tickets that he wanted. I agreed and began looking around. A man who heard that I wanted to trade tickets came to me saying, "My wife and I have a cruise we aren't going to be able to use. We will give you our cruise for two people if you will give us two tickets to the Packer-Bears game." I didn't really need another cruise; after all, I am on the water just about half of my time, but I couldn't turn him down. We found the time, and off we went. It was on a Carnival ship that left from Miami. It only lasted four days, but it was fun to see what the really big ships were like.

When I was on one of the smaller sailing ships I had a rather large order of drugs and supplies come in. I had no nurse to help me with them, and we were taking on new passengers as I was unpacking them. I had to add them to the inventory and place them in a book that shows when they would be outdated, before placing them in their proper place. I had noticed that we had a bottle of Valium that was outdated, so we had ordered a bottle of 100 five-milligram tablets of Valium to replace them. They had arrived with the other things. During the course of the afternoon as I worked, I had left the infirmary door open. I noticed that a lady with two boys was moving into the cabin across the hall from the infirmary. Shortly after they were settled, she came in to the infirmary to let me know that she had a thirteen-year-old boy who had an allergy to peanuts. A little later a physician came in. He asked if I would show him our infirmary. I probably spent five to ten minutes with him. Then our lady from across the hallway was back. She wanted to know if her son should inadvertently ingest some peanuts, what would I do? I explained exactly what would happen. Another passenger dropped in to talk about her ankles, which had become swollen on the airplane ride to the ship. I think about two crewmen also came by with minor complaints during the afternoon. The lady from across the hall came in two more times with questions about her son.

I was finally finished with the supplies, and when I went to get the outdated bottle of Valium, I realized the new bottle of Valium wasn't there. I had checked it in, and it was now missing. I went right to the hotel manager and told him that the Valium had probably been stolen. He said that that was too bad, but there wasn't much we could do about it and he did not feel like we should report it any further. However, I did report it to Seattle. They immediately got back to the captain and wanted to know what was being done to find out what had happened. The captain came down to the infirmary and I told him about my suspicions that the lady across the hall had probably taken them. He said, "We can't accuse her because she was only one of several people who could have taken it, but we can sure check the crew quarters." So all the crew cabins were inspected. All the storage areas of the ship were checked. Nothing was searched where I thought it could probably be found. Finally the captain said, "Now where are the boxes your supplies came in?"

"They went to the incinerator room," I said.

He said, "Well, I'm going to put down on my report that the Valium probably got back into an empty packing box and were lost in the packing material and now have probably been incinerated." I still think that woman got away with my Valium! After that, the infirmary door was always closed and locked when I was unpacking supplies.

We were going to go from Valparaiso, Chile, around

Cape Horn, stopping at the Falkland Islands, and then on to Buenos Aires and up the coast, ending at Fort Lauderdale. Punta Arenas is located on the Straits of Magellan. There is a large statue to the Patagonian Indians located in Punta Arenas. Patagonia means big foot, and the statue has an Indian with a very large foot sticking out. Where the big toe is located, it can easily be reached. Legend has it that if you rub the toe, you will live to return to Punta Arenas in good health. I didn't believe I would ever be there again, but I rubbed that toe vigorously! A year later I was back. I rubbed it again and maybe someday I'll be able to get there again.

As we rounded Cape Horn, I expected bad weather, but there wasn't any. The temperature was fifty-six degrees, the wind was at six knots and the sea was relatively calm. We stopped the ship and watched the penguins playing around it. There is a weather station on Cape Horn and a huge statue of an albatross to honor all the sailors who died while they were going around the Cape. We proceeded on to the Falkland Islands just in time to see Prince Charles, who was visiting the island for the first time!

We heard of a large rookery for penguins, located about five miles from Stanley, the capital city. We caught a cab out and the cab driver assured us that he would leave us for one hour and then return again. I told him that I would wait to pay him when he came back to pick us up. The beach in that area had been booby trapped during the war with Argentina. The mines could be set off by the weight of a man, but not by the weight of a penguin. The mines had not been removed, and the penguins had taken over the area that was undisturbed by humans. Nobody was going to go there. It was a very interesting area. We were back to the agreed meeting place well before the hour was up. No cab. An hour and a half went by. Still no cab. Two hours, and we were about to start walking when another cab came along—not the one that had brought us out to see the penguins. We explained our predicament to the driver and he said he would take us back to town. He then asked if we had paid the other driver and I said "no."

He said, "Then I'll charge you for a round trip and I will see that he gets his money for bringing you out."

I don't believe for one minute that he gave money to the other cab driver, but it was well worth the price to get back to the ship on time.

We were sailing along the western coast of Costa Rica. We stopped at an inlet where there was a beautiful beach, three or four houses, and a jungle right in back of the houses. I was told that Howler monkeys were common in this area and I decided to walk back into the jungle to see if I could see any. I walked along a dirt road for a little while. I then turned onto a foot path. I soon caught up with an older female passenger who was hiking along, also hoping to see monkeys. I passed her and she continued to follow me probably twenty or thirty feet behind. I came to a clearing and as I looked up, I could see monkeys in the tree tops. I stopped and watched them play. The passenger, who saw me stop, also stopped. I was in the clearing and she was under a coconut palm tree on the edge of the clearing. As I watched, a monkey crossed to the palm tree and began to pick the coconuts and throw them at the lady. She jumped back away from the tree with a loud scream. The monkey ran and so did she!

I write postcards, from many of the ports I visit, to my children, grandchildren, sisters, and cousins, and some people who just like to hear from me. We were in Granada once and I went to the ship's front desk to get fifteen stamps for my fifteen cards. I was told, "We don't have any local stamps, but just leave your cards with us along with a dollar a card and we will give them to the port agent who will stamp and mail them." I did but he didn't. No one that I had sent cards to received them. He obviously pocketed the money and discarded the cards. The next time I was in the eastern Caribbean, I made up my mind that I would go to the local post office and buy stamps and apply them myself. I had my cards written out when we reached the island of Guadeloupe. Guadeloupe is French. I inquired as to the location of the post office and found it to be within walking distance. There were probably five or six people in line waiting to buy stamps. I joined the line. When it was my turn, I held up my cards, pointed to the American addresses and then pointed at the stamps. The postal worker picked up the cards and counted them, and then counted out fifteen stamps. Then I handed her American money. She immediately grabbed the stamps back and pushed my money back to me. I reluctantly took my cards back and turned to leave. There was a middle-aged man standing behind me. He stepped forward, and at the same time took my cards. He proceeded to pay for the stamps in francs. Then I tried to hand him my American money, but he declined to take it. What a wonderful gesture! What a wonderful French man!

Saba is one of my favorite Caribbean Islands. It has a large inactive volcano and about 5,000 residents. The main city is located in the bottom of a central crater. They have named the city "The Bottom." They have a road that leads around the island to the other side, where there is a small village. The road is paved with concrete that the villagers mixed and poured themselves. There are several signs with the name "The Road," and of course the village is called "The Other Side." One side of the mountain goes up high into the air. They have cut steps into the side so that they can climb to the top for the view, and this mountain is called "Mount Scenery." The main industry on the island is a medical school.

It was 1999. A 2000 Wish List had just come out. I was sailing to Alaska. Nancy Ellis was one of my nurses and she announced that she had confirmation that she would be one of the nurses on the 2000 world cruise. She suggested that I should also ask to go on it. I said that I wouldn't mind going, but I was sure that having gone on the World Cruise in 1997, I would never get it again. She said, "You sure won't get it if you don't ask!" She then went back in her office and set up the computer to contact Seattle, and said. "Now you do the rest." I hadn't seriously considered asking, but she was so insistent that I sat down at the computer and began to write. "I would like the 2000 World Cruise for several reasons. First, I'm experienced. I was on the 1997 World Cruise. Second, I'm available for the whole 96 days. Third, Nancy Ellis has just asked me to go along with her." I got an immediate answer back, "We can't make it official, but you're on." It is a long time to be on the water, but the first World Cruise was 103 days, so I pointed out to my wife that this one was much shorter, only ninety-six days! She still wasn't sure that she could take that many days on the water, but reluctantly she decided to go.

The time came to leave and this time we were starting at Fort Lauderdale and went south first, around South America, and then east. The last World Cruise went west and this direction is much easier because every time we moved fifteen degrees, we'd get an extra hour of sleep. So twenty-four nights out of the 103, you have one extra hour. When going east you lose one hour of sleep. Again, you get it back as an extra day when you cross the International Date Line. Just recently I came from Singapore to Los Angeles, and we had two Wednesdays that week as we crossed the Date Line. Of course I worked on both days. I get paid by the day and when I got my pay in Los Angeles, the purser hadn't paid me for the extra day. I pointed this out to her and she said, "Well, you got paid for a day you didn't work going the other way." I pointed out to her that I had flown to Singapore and I only wanted to be paid for the days that I had worked. She sat down with a calendar and I could tell she hadn't figured it out, but she still paid me.

We got settled on the *Rotterdam VI* and we had our own cabin this time. Again, there was a full complement of passengers, a number of whom we had sailed with in 1997. There was Mr. Weatherspoon, who was ninety-nine years old, and he was sailing on his thirty-fourth World Cruise! There was Kissing Annie. No one knew her age. She was a short, little old Jewish lady who was remembered for four things. First she came aboard the 1997 World Cruise with 103 outfits (so she could have a different change of clothing every single day). The second thing was she danced with all the men on the ship, and if they would try to escape her by saying they couldn't dance, she would insist on teaching them. Third, she would kiss any man or woman, anyone that she could possibly pull down to her height, which was something like four feet eight inches. Fourth, she would always take in the evening entertainment. She would take a chair from the back of the lounge and drag it down into the very first row, sit down, and go to sleep!

Our first stop was Grand Cayman Island where Rachel shared a cab to Hell with Mr. Weatherspoon. Hell is an area in the center of the island where the black coral formations are exposed. From there we went on through the Panama Canal and down the west coast of South America. We stopped in Ecuador, which is where the Panama hat is made. So it was off to a market for Rachel and me. She was a little worried about carrying her billfold and decided to slip a little money into her glasses case. She was wearing sunglasses, and her brand new prescription lenses that she had just purchased before our trip were in the case with her money. At the end of the day as the sun was getting low, she took off her dark glasses, and reached into her bag to discover that someone had stolen the glasses case. There wasn't much money left in it; she had spent most of it during the day. But she felt badly about losing her new glasses.

There's always someone on board the ship to lecture people about what to expect at the next port. Our next port was the one that would give us access to Lima, Peru. The port lecturer finished his lecture by saying, "Now don't wear any expensive jewelry or watches into Lima. We don't want to invite theft." Having said that, he caught a cab into Lima that had no air-conditioning, so he had his window open and was sitting with his arm on the windowsill at a stop light. And, of course, someone grabbed his expensive watch off of his arm! To my knowledge, he was the only one who lost anything in Lima.

Further on down the coast of South America we stopped at General San Martin. This is a port that is ten miles from the town of Pisco, Peru. I took a public bus into town and I got off the bus at about noon at a town square in the middle of the town. I started walking down a street where there were a number of colorful street vendors. I was taking lots of pictures and I didn't realize that I had wandered probably five or six blocks from the town square. A police car pulled up alongside me and there were four policemen in it. One jumped out with an automatic weapon in his arms and started speaking rapidly in Spanish! I didn't understand one word and I told him so with gestures. Then he proceeded to grab my camera and act like he was going to run off with it. Then he motioned for me to turn around and go back the way I had come. His message was clear and I rapidly turned and started toward the city square. The police car also turned around and it followed me all the way back to the square. I didn't leave the square until the next bus came along, and then it was back to the ship for me.

We proceeded south to Arica, Chile. This area is located almost on the border between Peru and Chile and is dry. It hadn't rained there in fourteen years. We were going to visit the world's driest golf course. The average annual rainfall on the golf course was .014 inch. There were trees there that were largely piles of rocks painted green with an occasional dead palm tree that someone had stuck into the sand. And there were water hazards—these were piles of rocks painted blue. Everyone carried a piece of green carpet that they would place on the sand. Then they would place their ball on the carpet in order to facilitate hitting it.

We rounded Cape Horn. This time there was more of what we would expect to see with gale force winds—probably less than one-quarter mile visibility. It was entirely different than the last time we were there. I understand now why there is no vegetation on Cape Horn—the wind blows it away.

Then we dropped down to Antarctica. This is the world's driest continent, the world's windiest continent, and the world's coldest continent. We sailed along the coast of Antarctica for about two days. The weather was perfect for the first one-and-a-half days and I took several hundred pictures of the breathtaking rugged beauty with huge icebergs created by the breaking up of the shelf ice. We had some stormy weather as we left the area and turned to the north. The next morning the captain came on the intercom and said, "I think you should know that as we were crossing Drake's passage last night, we had ninety-five mile per hour winds. Those are hurricane force winds." I had slept right through them, so I had no idea what they had done, if anything, to the ship.

We headed up to Buenos Aires. I had always wanted to see Iguaso Falls, situated way up on the Argentine/Brazilian border. But despite having been in South America several times, I hadn't made it there yet. I was determined this time that I would. We were to be in Buenos Aires two days, which would give Rachel and me a chance to fly there for a day. Iguaso Falls consists of 256 separate water falls. All are two times the height of Niagara Falls. The volume of water that goes over those falls is larger than any falls in the world. It supplies the power for northern Argentina, southern Brazil and all of Paraguay. I spent the day hiking along the bottom of the falls, and then up on the top where you get the best view of the many rainbows. It was truly an unforgettable sight.

I loved Cape Town, South Africa, with table Mountain, which has cloud cover that some call "God's tablecloth." We went on to Madagascar, and that is a very unusual island, but a very poor island. It probably had the poorest economy of any of the places we visited on this trip.

Kenya was another high point. We anchored at Mombasa, and we took a day-long trip out to the savannah to visit Tsavo National Park and see the animals. On the way, we stopped for a bathroom break. I took one look at what they called a bathroom and decided I'd wait! I felt it couldn't get any worse.

I was wearing my Panama hat that I had bought for one U.S. dollar in Ecuador, using it to shade myself from the sun. A native approached me and asked if I would trade my hat for two hand-carved elephant bookends. I did, and later I gave them to my grandson. We stopped at a Masai village on the way back. The head nurse asked me to take her picture with one of the colorfully dressed natives, and as I did, she slipped her arm around him. That was a mistake. She was scratching bites for the next two or three days. We stopped next at the Seychelle Islands off the coast of Kenya. I had always felt that the beaches of Virgin Gorda in the Caribbean, with rock formations called "The Baths," were among the most beautiful beaches in the world. But the Seychelles have beach areas that are even more beautiful.

When we got into Thailand, we did one of the things most tourists do—go for an elephant ride. I made arrangements for Rachel to do that with me. Her first response was, "No way are you going to get me up on an elephant!" I reminded her that when we were in India, she rode on elephants up the side of a mountain, and she said, "But I'm older." A year before, she had had hip replacement surgery, so she said, "And what if I would fall off the elephant? I would probably break my artificial hip, and maybe I'd break the good one too!" I explained to her that this ride was on level ground. They had a platform that you walked on to get onto the elephant with two men to assist you, and likewise there's a platform to help you get off with the assistance of two men, and of course a knowledgeable driver sitting on the front of the elephant's head. Very reluctantly, she went. When she saw that everything I had said was true, she got on that elephant and away we went. At one point our driver slid off the elephant and suggested that I might want to take over in guiding it, but I assured him I was just along for the ride and I had no interest at all in taking over his job. He took some pictures of us and then he got back on. We concluded our ride and returned to the ship.

As we were approaching the dock, I noticed that there was an ambulance sitting nearby, and the other doctor, who was on call while I was out riding elephants, was standing nearby. I went over to him and asked what he had in the ambulance and he said, "It's a broken hip." And I asked, "How did it happen?" He said, "She fell off an elephant!" It turned out that the passenger weighed nearly 300 pounds, and as she was stepping off the elephant with the help of the two assistants, the elephant stepped away from the stand and she stepped right down between the elephant and the stand. There was no way those two little Thais could stop her fall. She ended up going back to the States for repairs.

Rachel had several nephews who had served in Vietnam and she was eager to see the country. She signed up to take a shore excursion to Ho Chi Minh City. The morning of the excursion arrived and I was on duty until noon and wouldn't be going with her. About half an hour after she was supposed to have gone, she came into the infirmary in tears. The Vietnamese security guards wouldn't let her get off the ship. Her papers were not in order. A port lecturer who had talked about Vietnam had said that not only do they change the rules of the game from day to day there, but they even change the goalposts. By afternoon, when I was off duty, we managed to get things worked out. We found a cab to take us out to see the surrounding area. When we were leaving the dock area, our cab was stopped by the police and I think when all was said and done, the driver had to bribe them in order to be allowed to take us out.

We stopped for a couple of days in Hong Kong. When we had been there last, it was under the control of England, and now it was part of China. It was interesting to see the changes. The very first things I noticed were the street signs. Before, all the street signs were in English with very small Chinese characters under large English words. Now they were all changed to large Chinese characters, with small English words underneath. All the police were in pairs. One spoke English and the other spoke Chinese.

We went on to mainland China and visited the Great Wall for the second time. We visited the section of the wall that is located near Beijing, and my, how it had changed. There was now a charge to walk on the wall, and the people on the wall were mainly foreigners. Before that, there would have been literally hundreds of Chinese enjoying the famous wonder.

We made a brief stop in Korea and then went on to a number of ports in Japan. At almost every port we were met by famous drummers, who wore masks while pounding vigorously on drums of every size. In Japan I was introduced to sweet potato ice cream and it didn't taste too bad.

It was the middle of the night when we were one day out of Japan. I was awakened by a tremendous BANG! It felt like we had been hit by another ship. Rachel had picked up an elephant when we were in Kenya. It was hand carved and about twelve inches long, and she had placed it on a shelf above our bed. With the bang, the elephant flew off the shelf and landed on my head. We learned later that we had been hit by a rogue wave. The side of the ship was dented in at approximately thirty-five feet above the water line. The metal deck in that area was bent up, along with the ribs going around the ship. We had welders on board from Honolulu to Los Angeles making temporary repairs, and eventually we needed to go into dry dock to make the final repairs. The power of the ocean is hard to believe.

About two days out of Japan, we had a gentleman with a coronary occlusion. Shortly after having his heart attack, he developed a third-degree heart block. Then a second man had his kidneys shut down. We really needed to get both of these men to a hospital. We discussed the situation with the Coast Guard and they said there was a good airfield at Midway Island. Midway Island was a refueling stop during World War II, and after the war it was turned into a national bird sanctuary. The permanent population was limited to 130 people, and until recently, tourists were not allowed to stop there. Now there are 175,000 pairs of albatross on the island, and they are known as "gunney birds." Because of the birds, planes are not allowed to land during the daytime, but they may land at night when the birds were resting. The coastguardsmen said they would try to get special permission to land during the day, and if they could, they would send a C-130 from San Diego to pick up our patients and take them to Honolulu.

The day arrived and the wind and the waves were too high for us to go into port. So the Coast Guard sent out a cutter to retrieve my two patients and me. We had the patients strapped into basket-type stretchers. The boat pulled up alongside our ship and was making five-foot excursions up and down beside us. I had two small bags: one with medications for the patients and one with a few clothes and my camera. As the Coast Guard vessel was going up and down, I passed my bags to the sailor who then threw them into a small cabin behind him. Then he grabbed me and I found myself on the deck. To get to the cabin there was a small companionway that turned sharply. It was impossible for us to take our patients inside so I found a somewhat protected area on the open deck and placed the patients there. The Coast Guard had two basket-type stretchers and I transferred one of my patients from our basket to theirs. But when I checked on the second basket, it was all wet and I decided to continue to use our basket. We got to the shore and I transferred the patients to an ambulance. I reached for my camera because there were birds everywhere. But my camera was broken. It would not take

141

pictures. So here were 175,000 pair of birds and I don't have a picture of one of them!

The plane was waiting for us on the runway, which was covered with birds. The local water supply comes from rain that falls on the runway, and there are no wells. I couldn't help but wonder what it would take to purify the water before I'd be willing to drink it. The airplane was well equipped and we quickly transferred our patients to cots on board the plane. The pilot warned us that we probably would have bird strikes upon taking off and to be prepared for almost anything! We were very quickly airborne. We could see the birds on every side but I don't believe we did too much damage to the bird population. It was a smooth flight and we arrived in Honolulu at about midnight, and transferred our patients to the hospital uneventfully.

All of my staff had teased me, saying I had taken a two-day vacation while waiting for the ship to reach Honolulu—two full days of lying on the Waikiki Beach. I awakened the next morning to a rainstorm and in the next thirty hours we received three inches of rain. I was told that there was a large mall about two blocks from my hotel and I could probably get my camera fixed there. I had no umbrella and no raincoat, so I waited until I thought the rain had let up a bit and I started for the mall. It started raining again just as hard as before. My first purchase at the mall was an umbrella. I found the camera store and was informed that it would take two weeks to repair. I said, "Isn't there anywhere in Honolulu where I can find someone who will repair it right now?" The employee gave me an address of a place within walking distance, so I started off in the rain—but this time I had an umbrella. I waded through spots where the water was a couple of inches deep. I found the store, the repairman was there, and he had my camera fixed and working within five minutes!

When I got back to my hotel, I decided to call Mr. Weatherspoon. When we were in Japan, ninety-nine year old Mr. Weatherspoon had developed pneumonia. I had to leave him at a hospital in Japan. He was put on a floor where there were no English-speaking doctors or nurses. He immediately called Flight for Life in Honolulu and they agreed to send a plane for him at a cost of $90,000! So now he was in Honolulu. I called him and he said, "Am I glad to hear from you! I am well and ready to board the ship when it gets in here, and now you can make all the arrangements for me to do this." The first thing I did was call his doctor who was surprised to hear me say that Mr. Weatherspoon was well. His pneumonia was better, but he had developed cellulitis in both legs and was getting IV antibiotics. I told him we could handle the IV antibiotics but he would have to be able to dress himself and stay in his own room or we would not want him back on the ship. When the doctor made rounds, he was met with a smiling, fully dressed Mr. Weatherspoon, all ready to check out. He said, "See? I can care for myself!"

The ship came and the first words my staff said to me were, "Where is our stretcher basket?" It was the first time that I had thought about it.

I said, "I think it's probably on Midway Island." I was told that the basket was practically new and had cost 600 dollars.

My staff said," "You left it on Midway Island?" I did, and I was told that after several months, someone did ship it to Seattle and HAL got it back.

Mr. Weatherspoon had his legs wrapped in Ace bandages. He didn't want them on at night. He said, "I can take them off, but I can't put them back on in the morning." "No problem," I said, "come on down to the clinic in the morning. When we give you your IV antibiotics, I'll put them back on for you." The very first morning that he came down, he had forgotten to bring the Ace bandages with him. I said, "No problem. We have a lot of Ace bandages here. I'll just sell you some new ones." He wanted to know how much the new ones would cost. When he heard that they would probably cost $8 apiece, he said, "No way! You're going to send someone up to my room to get my old, perfectly good Ace bandages." Here's a man who had just paid $90,000 because he didn't like the Japanese language!

When we got to Los Angeles, I wanted to put Mr. Weatherspoon back in the hospital again. He said, "I'm scheduled to go to Fort Lauderdale; that's where my car is, and I'm not getting off on the west coast." However, he did get off. Before he left, he put a 500-dollar deposit down for the 2001 World Cruise. I understand that he never sailed again. He died several months after I last saw him.

The five days from Hawaii to Los Angeles proved to be very busy because of an attempted suicide. Shortly after the start of the world voyage, a lady of about thirty-six years of age came into the infirmary. She said that she was a sixth-grade teacher, and had slipped and fallen at work, injuring her knee. She also said that she was completely disabled. She wanted me to write a letter on a weekly basis to her insurance company saying that she continued to be totally disabled. This was in order for her to receive disability compensation during the world voyage. I said, "You walked in here at the start of world voyage, no crutches, not even a cane, very little limp and you want me to say that you are completely disabled?" I told her that I would be happy to write her insurance company to tell them that she was on board and recovering nicely. I didn't see her again until the night after we had left Hawaii. She had been found on her bathroom floor unconscious, in shock and barely breathing.

Her troubles began when she was a teenager. She had a stepfather who sexually abused her. She told her mother what was happening, and her mother said that if something inappropriate had happened then she must have encouraged it. She felt completely abandoned by her mother and left home to live with an aunt for a number of years. During that time she had absolutely nothing to do with her mother. Her stepfather died and her mother was anxious to make things right with her. Her mother thought this world cruise might be helpful in repairing their relationship. Her knee injury would allow her time off from her teaching job and she accepted her mother's invitation. They did not get along on the trip, and when we were in Hawaii she took her mother's credit card and made multiple purchases with it. Her mother was upset.

In the course of their argument, the daughter said, "I might just as well commit suicide."

Her mother replied, "Go ahead! Good riddance of bad rubbish!" And then she went to bed. The daughter consumed half a bottle of Jack Daniels, thirty five-milligram Valium tablets, and twenty Vicodin. Her mother got up to use the bathroom during the night and found her nearly dead daughter lying on the bathroom floor. She was comatose for two days. We needed to give her medications to combat the Vicodin and neutralize the effects of the Valium, and we needed to keep her blood pressure up with Dopamine. When she finally awoke, she was very angry and combative! She was angry with her mother, angry with us, and angry with the world in general. In part, this was because as she was waking up, we had to keep her in restraints. She was not happy with the fact that we had saved her life. When we reached Los Angeles she was the first one off the ship for her continued psychiatric care.

When the 2001 Wish List came out, I noticed there was one voyage in October that started in Istanbul, Turkey, that stopped in Tel Aviv and Haifa, Israel, and then proceeded on to Tampa, Florida. I asked for the assignment and got it. We made arrangements to go early for this particular assignment in order to spend four extra days in Israel. I had still never been to Israel in spite of being assigned twice to ships that were supposed to stop there but for various reasons didn't.

Then came 9/11. The travel company in Chicago that was making our hotel reservations in Israel called us. They first said, "Why do you want to go to Israel?"

I said, "Merely to see the Holy Land."

They said, "That's not a good enough reason. We no longer are making any reservations for tourists."

In October we went and picked up our ship in Istanbul, Turkey, but they had eliminated Haifa, Tel Aviv, and Alexandria from their itinerary. They added several of the Greek islands and the west coast of Greece and Corsica to the scheduled stops. Just before 9/11 we had spent a month on the *Windspirit* in the Aegean Sea. We went from Istanbul to Athens and back, and we spent time on several of the Greek islands along the way. Several interesting things happened during that time.

We were sailing down the middle of the Aegean Sea. When we sail without using our motors, all is quiet, and there is no engine vibration. It was fifteen minutes before midnight and I was asleep. Someone came knocking at my door and said, "We have a man overboard. Go to the lifeboats." When I got to the lifeboat deck, our tender was approaching. I learned that as we sailed along, several of the crew members and passengers had heard screaming coming from the water. The sails are computer operated and we quickly rolled them up and reversed the engines, lowered a tender, and found two men in the water. We had almost hit them and we never would have heard them if we had been in one of HAL's larger ships. One was a native of Afghanistan and one was a Shi'ite Moslem from Turkey. They were seeking political asylum in Greece and had left Turkey at sundown in an inflatable kayak. They had put their clothing in a garbage bag to keep it dry and had started out in shorts and life jackets. The kayak developed a leak and sank. They had been in the water about three hours. They were quickly brought on board. I took them down to the infirmary. They were shaking more from fear than from the water because the water wasn't all that cold. Their temperatures were normal. I put them in bed to help control the shaking. We called the chief housekeeper who managed to round up some old uniforms to give them, and we called the kitchen staff and they sent up some pizzas. We got ahold of the Greek authorities, and to the captain's surprise, they agreed to come out to the ship and pick up the men.

The next voyage on the *Windspirit* was going to be a private trip. Two men had chartered the ship. One was a spiritual intermediary who had written several books. One was a psychologist who was also a hypnotist. He, too, had written several books, and had been on radio and television. Both had a following. They had invited this following to join them in an attempt to contact loved ones who had passed over. Many of them also wished to get in contact with their former lives. We met a couple from New Jersey. The wife was Swiss and the husband was from the Bronx. The wife was a strong believer in what she was experiencing on the ship. The husband attended the spiritual meetings to please his wife but felt they were all a hoax. We had good-natured arguments about religion and the difference between the views that they held and the more fundamental views that Rachel and I held. Shortly before they disembarked, the husband said, "Now my wife and I had an audience with the Pope and then we had a second audience that included our children. Each time we were given a rosary blessed by the Pope. We were also given holy water that had been blessed by the Pope." He continued, "Now I know you folks are sincere religious people and I wonder if you would like one of our rosaries and a little of the holy water." I said I thought that was very kind of them to want to share the water with us. We parted ways. This was just before the events of 9/11 occurred and I quickly forgot our conversation.

Not long after 9/11, the anthrax scare was in all the papers. Certain items were listed that we should be very careful with. Any envelopes with too much postage, any letters with block printing, particularly if they were from someone who you did not know, and any letters from New Jersey. We were told to be suspicious of any one of those things. There was a note on our door that said the post office had tried to deliver mail to us when we were not home, so we should pick it up at the post office. When I went in to pick up the mail, the postal clerk shoved an envelope across the counter in my direction. The very first thing that I noticed was that there was twelve dollars and fifty cents postage on the envelope. The address was printed in block letters; it was postmarked from New Jersey, and the return address was from someone I didn't know. I asked the postal clerk if she'd seen any white powder spill out of the envelope and she said, "Oh, no, no! It's well sealed!" I took it home unopened. As I looked at the name, it began to dawn on me that this could be from the people that we had met on the ship. I went ahead and opened the envelope. There was no anthrax, just our promised holy water and rosary!

What happened to my holy water? I hadn't heard from Dottie in several years. She was the secretary who worked for me early in my practice in De Pere and volunteered to work short term for me when I was desperately trying to find satisfactory help at the close of my practice. When we were in Florida, out of the blue, I received a phone call from Dottie. She wanted me to know that she had just had a colon resection for a primary cancer of the colon. At that time she was fifty-six years old. The tumor had extended into the adjacent tissue. Five months later she noted a lump in her right breast, which proved to be a new primary carcinoma.

Dottie had two daughters and a son. Her son Steve was studying to be an actor. Her older daughter, Maggie, was married with children and was a real comfort to her mother. Her younger daughter, Katie, had become involved with drugs. In order to support her habit, she had turned to stealing. She had stolen from Dottie and her husband, and when this was not enough money to support her habit, she became involved in prostitution. She had found a black man who was acting as her pimp. She had been picked up by the police and was now in jail. She had just told Dottie that she was pregnant with her pimp's child.

Back to the holy water! On the day that it arrived, Dottie called me to tell me that she suspected that Steve was bulimic and that the court had just called her and asked for her to testify against her daughter. It was evident that Dottie was depressed. Dottie is a devout Catholic and I offered to give her my holy water. That afternoon I dropped it off at her house along with thirty Prozac capsules. Did it do any good? I don't know. What I do know is that Dottie has no evidence of any recurrence of either tumor, that

Steve is finished with school and has successfully started in his chosen career, and that Katie is out of jail and is giving lectures on drug rehabilitation.

We were on our way back to Fort Lauderdale after sailing in the Caribbean when a Dutch lady came into the infirmary. She spoke little English. I was informed that she was a neighbor of our hotel manager, who was also from Holland. She had a history of gallstone colic, and I thought there was a good chance that she had perforated either her gallbladder or her stomach. I felt that she should promptly have exploratory surgery on her abdomen.

Our next port destination was Half Moon Key, a private island owned by Holland America. The island was thirty-six hours away. I asked the captain if we were passing by any island where we could have her transferred to Miami. He said, "Keep her on board until we reach Half Moon Key." I decided to call the Coast Guard. They had been so helpful to us at Midway Island. I talked with the Coast Guard surgeon on duty and he agreed that we should promptly get her to Miami for surgery. He asked if he could talk with the captain. He stayed on the line while I got the captain to come down to the infirmary. He wanted to know our exact location. Then he pointed out to the captain that at four P.M. we would be passing a little island that had an airstrip. It also had one doctor, and the Coast Guard would be able to pick up our patient at approximately six P.M. Everyone agreed that would be a good arrangement and we decided that our crew doctor would go ashore with the patient. I asked him to take his passport and some money with him and told him that if he had any concerns about the facility where we were leaving her, that he should stay with her. He came back to the ship and said, "Everything will be just fine for that two hours that she will be there.

The doctor on the island agreed to look after her until the Coast Guard takes over."

The next morning I received a call from the hotel manager. He wanted to find out how his neighbor was doing and he had decided to call her son, who was back in Holland. Her son had said, "She's still on the island!" I started calling *everyone* who was involved. The Coast Guard, when they found out that she was Dutch, decided that they couldn't pick her up because they were not on American territory. They considered her a foreigner on foreign soil. The last time I had used the Coast Guard, it was on Midway Island, which is American, and both patients had also been American. Instead of letting us know, they had called a private carrier in Miami and asked them to go and pick her up. This carrier called her husband and asked for credit card numbers. He gave them two, but when they checked the cards, the cards could not be charged for the 10,000 dollars that was needed to bring her to Miami. The carrier told the patient's husband that they weren't going to come for her until he could get the money together to send to them. No one bothered to let us know what was happening. We would've gladly vouched for the payment for her. We finally managed to get her to Fort Lauderdale for surgery. At the time of her surgery, a perforated duodenal ulcer was found. We had placed her on gastric suction and IV antibiotics, which were continued until her surgery, and she was actually improving during her stay on the island.

I was scheduled to meet the *Windsong* in French Polynesia the day after Christmas. Rachel had decided not to join me on this trip. She felt that too much was happening at home and she really didn't want to go at that time of year. Two weeks before leaving, I called to make my transportation arrangements. I said, "Stephanie, I need tickets to French Polynesia for December twenty-sixth."

"You haven't heard?"

"Heard what?"

"The *Windsong* caught fire at one A.M. yesterday and it is still burning! Everyone got safely off that night. It has now been sunk and is an artificial reef near Tahiti." Rachel was happy that I wasn't going to leave, but it made me very sad to think of the sinking of a ship that we had sailed on many, many times.

Within a day or two I got the official word that I wouldn't be needed in Tahiti. But, I was asked whether I would mind sailing out of Cape Canaveral for two weeks. We were there when the ill-fated *Columbia* took off. It was necessary for me to put one of our Indonesian crew members into the hospital while we were there. Security was so tight that I was informed we would have to pay to have a guard placed at his hospital room doorway to ensure that he did not leave his room. It was hard for me to believe that this was necessary.

I had been assigned to the MSY/SS *Windsurf*, the largest sailing ship in the world. We had over three hundred passengers and over one hundred ninety crew members. We were anchored at West Bay Beach on the island of Roatan, off the coast of Honduras, when Rachel and I decided to go to the village of West End. It was about a ten-minute trip by water taxi. The boat was small and we hit a few waves fairly hard, but we made it safe and sound. I could see Rachel talking to a cab driver who was sitting close to where we were exiting the boat. She had decided that she did not want to go back to our ship by boat and that we would take a cab instead. There were several small shops along the street that we started to visit. As we would exit each shop, there would be the cab driver asking if we were ready to go yet. We finally said, "Yes, take us back to our ship." Off we went. Only then did we realize that he spoke and understood very little English. He drove and drove, and the further he drove the more nervous Rachel became. As he continued to drive, I started wondering just what was happening. As we approached the town of Coxen Hole we saw a celebrity cruise ship. The cab driver indicated that this was our destination. I finally got through to him that this was not our ship. It was the wrong ship, and we wanted to go back to where he had picked us up. After fifteen kilometers of winding roads we found ourselves again at the village of West End but at a location that we were not familiar with. As we sat there pondering what to do, the cab driver called to a passing lady who spoke and understood a little more English than he did. We explained to her where our ship was located, but we were not sure that she understood us. Just as we were about to get out of the cab, off he went again. This time we managed to get to the right spot. A trip that should have taken about ten minutes actually took over ninety minutes.

Rachel stayed at the beach barbecue and I caught the tender back to the ship. There was a lady with a tooth abscess waiting for me, and the food and beverage manager had lacerated his finger cutting buns at the barbecue. As I was placing stitches in his finger, the loudspeaker came on and announced a "bright star" at the port side gangway. Bright star is the code word to get the medical team with all its emergency equipment together. I was the only member of the emergency team who was not at the beach barbecue on shore. I was told that the ship's hostess was involved in a serious accident. She had been on a shore excursion called The Canopy Tour. On this tour people go up into the trees and slide down a cable. Each person would be in a harness and would slide to a tree stand. This was repeated several times until the person finally reached the ground. As the hostess was descending on one of these cables she lost control and first ran into the operator, who was on the stand, and knocked him over. Then she hit the tree the cable was anchored to.

In order to get to the site of the accident, we took a dive boat from the ship to shore. Then we ran with all our equipment for about one hundred yards across the beach. Our emergency equipment consisted of an automatic external defibrillator, a small oxygen tank, and two boxes containing drugs and other equipment. A small truck was waiting for us. The truck drove at full speed for about three miles to the edge of a river. Here we got out and crossed the river on a narrow swinging bridge that was probably about one hundred yards long. It was supported by two cables, and it swung from side to side! Then we had to climb up a fairly steep hill for another two to three hundred yards. We arrived at the tree. Our patient was lying on a stand, about twelve feet in the air. Someone had produced a homemade ladder with one broken rung. It did not reach up to where the hostess was lying, but it did get me high enough so that I could take a few steps into the tree and then onto the platform. We managed to get a backboard under her. This was a difficult procedure because of the pain it caused her. Then she was lowered on the backboard by ropes. We carried her down a very steep hill to the waiting ambulance. I rode in the ambulance with her for fifteen kilometers to a little clinic. The clinic was clean, and on the surface seemed well equipped. However, the X-rays that they managed to take were all overexposed and almost unreadable. I thought we should not take her back on the ship, and we certainly couldn't leave her at the clinic. After calling our headquarters in Seattle, it was decided that we would have her evacuated by plane to a trauma center in Ft. Lauderdale. My only nurse came from the ship to stay with her until she could be picked up. The airport was not lighted, and the plane couldn't land at night. She was picked up the next morning. We learned that her injuries included the eleven fractured ribs, a broken seventh thoracic vertebra, and a broken left collarbone. It was three days before my nurse got back on board the ship—three whole days before I could set foot on dry land.

We had a chance to go on the MS *Princedam* toward the end of the year. The ship was going to visit Easter Island and Pitcairn Island. I had never been to either one and I felt that this was an opportunity that I couldn't pass up. When Stephanie from HAL's Seattle office was working on getting tickets for me to fly from West Palm Beach to Lima, Peru, she mentioned that my flight would come in to Lima at 11:30 at night. I pointed out to her that it usually takes about two hours from the airport until you are at the hotel and in bed, and that would be too short of a night to be on the ship by seven o' clock the next morning. She agreed and made our hotel reservations for two nights and flight arrangements for two days before the ship would sail. This was very unusual for HAL to do. Normally we fly in one day early because the ship can't sail without a physician on board, and that way we can still make the ship on time even if there is a delay in our flight. We arrived at our hotel at 1:30 in the morning. We cleaned up a bit and prepared to hop into our beds, only to discover that there were no sheets on my bed. The bed had been made with only the mattress cover underneath and the bedspread on top. I called the front desk and told the clerk that we needed sheets. Ten or fifteen minutes later there was a knock at the door, and there was a man with an arm load of blankets. Rachel was in her bed but I invited the man in and went over to my bed and turned down the bedspread to show him the mattress cover. Then I went to Rachel's bed and held up her sheets. He quickly exited the room, and after another ten or fifteen minutes he was there with two sheets. He went to the back side, and with me on the front side, we made the bed together.

It was nice to realize, as we got out of bed the next morning, that we had a day to spend any way we wanted. We went down to a little travel office in the front of the hotel and arranged for a city tour for that afternoon. I also learned that we were about six blocks from the Asian Market. The last time we were in Lima, we had visited the Asian Market. It is a complex of probably a hundred or more stalls that sell just about everything.

Last time we were in the Asian Market I had picked up a couple of framed sets of butterflies. There had been six or eight butterflies displayed under glass. I think they cost about six dollars each. We put them on the wall of my study in Wisconsin. Each time my son Terry came home, he would admire the butterflies and tell me to get some for him when I was back in Lima. When we were in Hawaii, my wife saw a similar set of butterflies and purchased them for Terry at a little over $100. She thought we would never get them at a bargain again and here we are six blocks from the Asian Market with a morning to spend there. One of the first things I saw displayed was butterflies. I couldn't get the price down below twenty-five dollars. I wanted one for my daughter, or for a wall in my study in Florida, or even for my next-door neighbors in Florida who have a butterfly garden between our house and theirs—if my daughter didn't want it then I would give to them.

In the meantime, Rachel had been looking at cards that had attractive pictures and were hand embroidered. She ended up not taking them. The one thing on our afternoon city tour that stood out in my mind was our visit to the Monastery San Francisco. There were catacombs under the cathedral where the dead had been buried. During a

156

three-hundred-year period, it was estimated that twenty-five thousand people had been buried there. There were six large round containers full to the top with bones, mainly long bones and skulls. Each were thirty-two feet deep and probably about twenty feet in diameter. The bodies were placed in boxes with one body on top of the next. Lime was placed between the bodies. When the flesh and small bones were gone, they would be transferred to the vats. It was a sight that I will never forget.

The next morning we were ready to go to the ship at 6:45 A.M. but no one came for us. I put in a call to the Port Agent and he told me that they were going to be unable to pick us up until eleven A.M. They had notified the shop but no one had bothered to tell us. When my wife heard that we weren't going anywhere, she suggested that maybe I would like to walk back to the market and get the cards she had been looking at the day before. I managed to arrive at the market at about 8:45 A.M. Everything was closed. I was ready to turn and leave when I noticed a tall Caucasian lady walking around the market area. I approached her and asked if she had any idea when the market opened. She said, "Oh, yes, anywhere from nine thirty to ten. Our hotel is just across the street, and I watch them open every day." It turned out that she was an American missionary and she was in Lima setting up a ten-step program for local alcoholics and drug-addicted residents of Lima. We talked for a half hour or so. I decided just to walk around the block until the market was open. At about 9:45 the stalls began to open and people were out sweeping and mopping the concrete in front of the stalls. At about ten o'clock I was able to get the cards my wife was looking for. As I was leaving the market, I noticed more butterflies, and also a display under glass of a large tarantula along with several bugs and worms. I asked for a price and was quoted fifteen dollars each. I picked up the butterflies and bugs, and handed the seller fifteen dollars. He said, "No, no. Twenty-five dollars for the two." When you really don't want something too much, it makes for good bargaining. I laid the frames down and reached over to take the money back from him. He hung on tightly to the money and put the butterflies and bugs into a plastic bag for me, and I headed back to the hotel.

Our first port of call after leaving Lima was General San Martin. This area is famous for the Nazca lines. These lines were constructed 2,000 years ago. They extend over 190 square miles. There is little rain in the area, and the prevailing winds keep the ditches that make up the lines free of dust. Upon leaving General San Martin, our ship passed by the Candelabra, which is the most famous of the lines. It sits on the side of a mountain. The ditches are six feet deep and six feet wide. They extended for thousands of feet, in perfect symmetry. No one knows just how it was accomplished.

We were on our way to Easter Island, which is the most remote island in the world. One must travel 1,178 miles from Easter Island to reach the nearest inhabited land. It was annexed to Chile in 1888. However, you must travel 2,300 miles to reach the mainland of Chile. Two days before arriving at the island, I was called to the infirmary to see a man who was having difficulty breathing. He had a history of three previous heart attacks and also coronary bypass surgery. We determined that he'd had pneumonia and then he had developed severe congestive heart failure. We started treatment, and at the same time started making arrangements for him to fly from Easter Island to a hospital in Santiago, Chile, for care until he could go to his home in Canada. With diuretics and antibiotics he improved enough so that I felt he would be able to fly commercially to Chile. We were scheduled to anchor at Easter Island at seven A.M. The airplane out was scheduled for 12:30 P.M. The morning of our arrival came, and when I looked out the porthole, we were traveling around the island at what appeared to be full speed. Two hours went by before it could be determined what had gone wrong and the engines could be slowed down. We were finally able to drop anchor and the port authorities came on board. They told us that the Santiago hospital suspected that our patient might have SARS (Severe Acute Respiratory Syndrome) and we must take our patient to the local clinic for them to rule this out before he could proceed on to Santiago.

The first tender came alongside the ship. As we attempted to get on board, the tender was making four to five foot excursions up and down the side of the ship. We would wait until the opening into the tender was at the same level as the opening into the ship, and then very quickly we would pass over into the tender. There was a very small ambulance waiting for us at the dock. When I managed to get my patient and his wife into the ambulance, the two ambulance attendants climbed into the front seat, and there was no room for me. I told my patient that I wouldn't be going with him in the ambulance and this was very upsetting for him, but fortunately the Assistant Port Agent picked me up shortly after and I was off to the hospital behind the ambulance. It had been raining for a week and there was red mud everywhere.

We arrived at a low-frame building that had a small waiting area. There were four beds in a larger room right next to the waiting area. The beds were separated by curtains for privacy. The building inside and out was in need of painting. The red mud had been tracked all over the room. Waste material was lying in the corners where it appeared to have been swept. After one glance I said to myself, I will never leave my patient here. If they won't release him to go to Santiago, then he will go back to the ship.

I was introduced to a man who obviously spoke no English and understood no English. Since my Spanish is poor, the only word of his that I recognized was the word "doctor." The Assistant Port Agent came to my rescue. He relayed my explanations about why this man couldn't possibly have a case of SARS. The doctor checked the records from the ship. He looked at the chest X-ray we had taken. There was no light box so he just held the X-ray in the general direction of the nearest window. Then he phoned someone else. It was eleven A.M. and I was getting a little nervous. A middle-aged man in a slightly soiled white coat showed up. With the Assistant Port Agent as my interpreter, I went through all the explanations that I had given the first man. His response was that we should send the Assistant Port Agent to our patient's wife to get her Visa card. Just then a man came in who could speak and understand English well. He was the Port Agent. He was full of apologies for all the delays. He reassured me that the plane was about one hour late and our patient would be on it. I stayed right by the man in the white coat until he had phoned Santiago and had permission for our patient to be on the plane. We went back through the mud and back to the ship. I did all this without my camera. I had planned to go back to the island in the afternoon to take pictures. This proved impossible. The captain announced that it had become too dangerous for anyone to leave the ship and the crew was concentrating on getting the people who were on shore back on board again. There were many disappointed passengers, including my wife. She didn't get to go ashore. However, salesmen did bring souvenirs from the island to sell to the passengers who didn't get off the ship. Rachel did end up with a large T-shirt that says, in small letters on the back side, "Easter Island."

We sailed away from Easter Island on a Monday and arrived at Pitcairn Island on Thursday, Thanksgiving Day. We were traveling west. With each fifteen degrees of travel, the clock would be set back one hour. This had happened Thursday at two A.M. I was wide awake and out of bed an hour earlier than usual. It was about six A.M. when I went to eat breakfast. I looked out to check on the weather and could see in the distance what appeared to be a big rock.

Pitcairn Island has been made famous by at least five movies and possibly a dozen books. The HMS *Bounty* sailed from England in 1788 in search of breadfruit trees to take and plant in Jamaica. Captain Bligh was in charge of the ship and Fletcher Christian was his first mate. Mutiny occurred on their return voyage. Captain Bligh and eighteen of his sailors were set adrift in a small boat. Fletcher Christian returned to Tahiti, picked up twelve Polynesian ladies and six Polynesian men, and with them and eight mutineers, he went to Pitcairn Island to seek sanctuary. It was eighteen years before an American ship happened upon them.

As we approached the island, we could make out activity on shore. The highest point on the island is about 1,000 feet. Sitting on top of this point is a Norfolk Island pine tree. We were told that people climb this tree to look for approaching ships. Between seven and eight cruise ships visit the island each year and a supply ship will come every three to four months. Their entire economy is dependent on the sale of stamps and souvenirs to the tourists.

We dropped anchor and I could see their longboat leaving the shore. The total population now is fifty-four, and every able-bodied man, woman and child was in that longboat, which was forty-eight in number. The island is

161

one and three-quarter square miles, or about 1,200 acres. However, only 100 acres can be used for the production of farm crops. The longboat pulled up alongsides and they began to unload boxes, bags and baskets by the dozen. Our security officer had been instructed to check in each one individually. He gave them an identification card to scan them in, and when they departed the ship, they were scanned out. This was to be sure that no one was left behind. We didn't want any stowaways.

After watching the check-in for a time, I had to go to the infirmary to work. The mayor of Adamstown came in and announced that he was also the dentist and wondered if we had an X-ray machine in our dental unit. We assured him that we did. Then he said he had two people with him that he would like our on-board dentist to see. They were taken care of. Then he displayed a splinted wrist and said that he suffered from carpal tunnel syndrome and wondered how I would treat it. I told him that we would use a splint first, and if this didn't help then we would use surgery to free up the median nerve.

Then he said, "Would you do the surgery right now? The splint has failed." I had to tell him no, this wasn't something that I would do. Then he said, "Well, if you have another splint it would help me in keeping it clean, and maybe you could give me a few pain pills." I was told that the Adamstown doctor was on board our ship, so I told the mayor that if he would send his doctor down, I could give him some outdated drugs that we had.

A short time later a nice-looking bearded man with an Australian accent showed up. He had been sent by the New Zealand government to Pitcairn. This was his second term of two years. He was not an M.D. but a Physician's Assistant. He took care of all the islanders' needs, from delivering the babies to caring for the injuries that occurred from falls while gathering bird eggs from the cliffs. It turned out that he was also the Seventh-Day Adventist minister for the island.

The Seventh-Day Adventists had sent missionaries to the island many years ago. They found a group of Anglican people who were already worshiping on Saturdays. When they had gotten back to religion, they had decided to worship on Sundays but hadn't taken into consideration the extra day when they crossed the International Date Line. Without realizing it, they were using Saturday as their day of worship. I asked the minister how devout these people were. He said, "Well, they all have an Adventist heritage, but only about thirteen or fourteen show up for church. You would think that they would be eager for any diversion on their small island."

Tables were set up to display the handcrafted items and stamps. I wrote a few postcards, including one addressed to myself and I bought stamps, and applied them to the cards, and asked the islanders to mail them for me. They were happy to mail them but informed me that I should expect it to take three to four months for them to get to their destination. An announcement came at about one P.M. that our guests should be off the ship in half an hour. I stood outside my infirmary door and watched them load their longboat with cases of toilet paper, and a while pallet piled high with cases of pop, watermelon, and even a few cases of beer and wine. They gathered up the items that weren't sold, got into the longboat, and began to sing in perfect harmony, "In the Sweet By and By" as they started for their homes back on shore.

Our next destination, after we sailed away from Pitcairn Island, was French Polynesia. The first island that we were to stop at was the island of Moorea. In two days we would be there. It is an island in French Polynesia that is one of Rachel's favorites. It is located about ten miles from Tahiti. On the way, a seventy-two-year-old man came into the infirmary in a wheelchair pushed by his wife. His head was hanging down as though it was just too heavy to hold upright. As I looked into our waiting room, I could see that his skin was jaundiced. The nurse was busy, so I stepped out into the waiting room and brought him directly into my office, ahead of the other waiting patients. I asked him how long his skin had looked like this and he answered two days. His only complaints were profound weakness and no appetite. He had drunk alcohol excessively for years. He had stopped seven months before we met, because he felt that he was gaining too much weight. He was given a short course of Zocor for his cholesterol and the combination had caused his liver enzymes to go up. His doctor knew this, but gave him permission to go on this cruise. I thought he was having liver failure. We started making arrangements for hospitalization in Papeete. We would be passing Tahiti at 6:00 A.M. on our way to Moorea. We planned to let down one of our tenders and take him to shore, where an ambulance would meet us and take him to the hospital. His kidneys began to shut down. His blood pressure dropped to 90/40. His pulse slowed; even his temperature dropped to 96.5 degrees. I felt that the end was close. The transfer to the hospital went well. It was with considerable surprise the next morning that we received an e-mail saying that he was stable and he and his wife hoped that within two to three days they would consider sending him home. That night he died.

We arrived at Moorea at about nine A.M. The peaks of its extinct volcano are nothing less than stunning to look at. We spent a day traveling up into the mountains, through the fields of pineapples, and picking ginger blossoms that grow along the road. Our next day was going to be in

Papeete, Tahiti. We wanted to get together with our good friends Diana and Frank Augustin. We had first met Frank seven years earlier. At that time we had decided to go to the local church.

We were met at the door of the church by someone who spoke only French and Polynesian. He recognized that we were Americans and called two men over, who introduced themselves and said that they would interpret for us. We walked down to the very front row, and my wife and I and another gentleman sat down beside Frank. The minister spoke in French, and a second individual stood beside him. He was the interpreter for those in the audience who only spoke Polynesian. After hearing the service in French and Polynesian we would then hear it in English. This was not our first experience listening to a French church service. We were in Iles des Saints in the Caribbean on Christmas Day once and there was a small Catholic church near where we had docked. We decided to go to the Christmas service there, and it was all in French with no interpreter. We didn't understand the words but we loved the music.

We became good friends with Frank and his family and we would plan to see them each time that we were back on the island of Tahiti. Rachel had written to Frank to say that we were coming. The day before our arrival, we had tried to phone them by satellite phone, but we were unable to make a connection. The morning came and there was no Frank. There is a tourist office near our dock and they were very helpful in contacting Frank where he worked. Frank teaches mathematics at a Seventh-Day Adventist college on the island. Their colleges correspond with our high schools. What we call college, they call university. Before long, there was Frank carrying a beautiful flower arrangement composed of Bird of Paradise, orchids, and other tropical blossoms. Traveling at his side was his seventeen-month-old son Mark. He placed shell leis around our necks, and we were able to spend the afternoon renewing our friendship. We spent four days on islands that were part of the Society Islands group. Then we went on to Christmas Island.

We arrived on Christmas Island on December 6. I felt that it would be something special if we were to send out our Christmas cards from Christmas Island. We learned that postage from the island to the States would be one dollar for each card and it would take eight weeks for delivery. My sister in West Palm Beach volunteered to mail our cards out instead. Christmas Island is the largest coral atoll in the world. The government is now independent, but it belongs to the British Commonwealth of Nations. In the 1950s the British used the island to test their nuclear bombs. The island was discovered by Captain Cook on Christmas Eve 1777. The average elevation of the island is ten feet, and the average rainfall is thirty inches. It is close enough to the equator so that nights and days are of equal length all year long.

The day we were there, sunrise was at 4:32 A.M. and sunset was at 4:32 P.M. The reason they are so early is because Christmas Island wanted to be the first place on earth to enter the new century on New Years Eve, so they adjusted their time zone to make it happen. The island is also famous because *Apollo 13* splashed down nearby when it came back from the moon. We had to tender in at Christmas Island. To tender in means that we don't dock, but we drop anchor and transfer everyone to shore by small boats. To find the way through the coral was very difficult, and we arrived at low tide, making it even more difficult. It was almost one P.M. before I reached the shore. I walked from the capital, which they call London, into the surrounding area, taking pictures of the thatched roof huts and the many happy children. There is even a sparsely equipped public library. I had gone about a mile when it suddenly started raining. I didn't mind getting wet but I hated to get my cameras wet. As I was looking for shelter from the rain, a car stopped and a young man said, "Could I give you a lift back to your tender?" I gladly accepted.

It had become a very busy cruise. There were increased cases of influenza Type A back in the United States and we were having our own little epidemic on board the ship. As we were approaching Honolulu, we received a call from a man claiming that he couldn't wake his wife. I had seen her four days before. At that time I had made the diagnosis of influenza. He claimed that she hadn't eaten anything and had drank very little during that four days. We brought her down to the infirmary and found out she was awake. However, she was disoriented and uncooperative. She didn't even know how old she was. Anything we would put in her mouth, she would spit out. She was septic and a very sick lady. We managed to get her into the hospital when we arrived in Honolulu. After leaving Christmas Island, we were going to spend four days on the Hawaiian Islands. Our first stop was going to be Honolulu.

In Honolulu we walked about three blocks from the ship to where we were able to catch a city bus to the International Market. The first time we went to the Hawaiian Islands was on a vacation in 1960. At that time we stayed for one week in the Moana Surfrider Hotel on Waikiki Beach. It was just across the street from the International Market. We asked our bus driver to call out the International Market when we passed by. He agreed to, but he didn't. One of the passengers told us when to get off.

The Market had grown but still looked much like I had remembered it from years before. The beach seemed much smaller because of the many hotels encroaching on it. On our first visit, the two main hotels were the Royal Hawaiian, which was still the same pink color, and the Moana Surfrider, with its huge banyan tree in the courtyard. I was to learn that the hotel was built in 1927 around this same large banyan tree and was the very first hotel on Waikiki Beach. Now there seemed to be a never-ending row of waterfront hotels. The Moana Surfrider was bigger and better. It was resplendent with Christmas decorations, model trains, and gingerbread houses. Gaily decorated trees were everywhere.

Kauai is known as the Garden Island. The hotels next to the water have spacious lawns and beautiful beaches, and are built up against a bank, with very little backyard. There was a law that said no building could be taller than the surrounding palm trees. By building next to the bank, they could go up as high as the palm trees that were on the top of the bank, so even the highest of the hotels were legal. We discovered that our cell phone worked in Hawaii, so Rachel was busy calling people when she wasn't out buying macadamia nuts!

In Nawilliwilli, a gentleman came in bleeding from his gastrointestinal tract. It was off to the hospital with him. Our last stop before sailing on to San Diego was Kona on the big island of Hawaii. During the day we were there we sent an asthmatic to the hospital. Our ship left port at about six P.M. At seven P.M. a very sick man came into the infirmary. He had a long history of chronic obstructive pulmonary disease. His heart was now failing and he had developed pneumonia secondary to influenza. I asked him, "Why didn't you come in before we had left the port?" and his answer was, "I was afraid that you would send me into the hospital." We had been underway about one hour. The captain agreed to turn the ship around and head back to port. It put us about four-and-a-half hours behind our schedule, but we would have five days to make it up. We were finally on our way to San Diego and, after that, home.

5

In Conclusion

May 17, 2003, was my seventy-sixth birthday. We had received an invitation to attend the wedding of Becky's oldest daughter, Katie, to be held on the same day. Becky, who had been so supportive in my practice through the years, now had four children. The youngest boy had been my last delivery. He was now seventeen years old. It hardly seemed possible, but seventeen years had gone by since I had last delivered a baby. As the wedding approached, Becky asked if I would act as the wedding photographer. Photography is my passion, but I had never acted as a sole photographer for a wedding before. With a little apprehension I accepted, and I arrived at the wedding a bit early. There were relatives waiting who I met and briefly spoke to. I mentioned that it was my birthday. It surprised me that everyone seemed to know this already. The wedding was beautiful, the bride was beautiful and the reception was in full swing when Katie got up in front and presented me with a birthday cake! I was really surprised and very honored.

After the wedding, I had lunch with Becky and we were discussing this book. She said, "You must tell the story about the gypsy lady who came into our office." I had <u>no</u> recollection of her until Becky began to talk about her. Becky had always had a remarkable memory, and she provided names and dates for many of the stories that I am telling in this book.

We have the Brown County fairground in the town of De Pere. House trailer parking is allowed in the fairgrounds and a group of gypsies were among those who once parked there. One middle-aged lady came into my office. I have no recollection of what her problem was, but I remember asking her what medication she was on. She replied, "Oh, I have them right here." She reached into the neck of her dress and pulled out two bottles of pills from her brassiere. I checked the bottles and then she redeposited them in her bra. When she left, she paid cash for her visit, which she also obtained from her brassiere. As she turned to leave, she reached into her bra and pulled out a pack of cigarettes, and as she went out the door, out came the lighter from the other side!

There's one more story that demonstrates Becky's remarkable memory. I had a young lady that was probably about eighteen years old who came for a complete physical examination. After completing her physical, she said that she had come in strictly so that she could get acquainted with me and I could get acquainted with her. She went on to say that she had learned that I had delivered her, and she was trying to find her birth mother. I assured her that I would try to help her. If I could locate her mother, I would let her know that her daughter was looking for her. Becky was able to tell me who the unwed mothers were that I had delivered during that period, and we were able to determine which individual was most likely the one. The father was a policeman from Chicago who had come to Green Bay for a Packer football game. It was a one-night stand. Her mother had moved from the area and I could not find her.

There is a lot of curiosity about my job as a cruise physician, and I will tell you just a few of the questions folks have asked me. I will also include some of my usual answers. 'When people die, what do you do with the body?

170

Do you bury them at sea?" No, we don't bury them at sea. HAL has a zero overboard policy. We had a lady die when we were sailing off the coast of Japan. We could not find any relatives, only a lawyer who seemed to be in charge of her affairs. When we explained to him what had happened, he said, "Well, she provided for that eventuality. If she died on this trip she asked to be buried at sea." We explained to him that this was impossible. We would be willing, however, to have her cremated in Japan and send her ashes back to him.

"How many caskets do you carry on board?" is another question I am asked. Now, a rumor went around that we always have five caskets on our world cruises. Untrue. We have no caskets on board. All the ships have modern morgues that will hold four bodies and keep the temperature just above freezing. The old *Rotterdam* stored bodies in the same refrigerator that the florist used for his flowers, but that is no longer the case.

"If you were ever to move from the United States, where would be your first choice to go?" That's easy; it would be New Zealand. New Zealand has a variety of climates, from the semitropical north, which has one of the most beautiful rose gardens that I have ever seen (located in Auckland), to the south, which is the jumping off place for many Antarctic expeditions. If your fancy is skiing, the Mount Cook area is a good place to be. New Zealand is not overcrowded at least not with people. I have heard that there are only three million people in all of New Zealand but there are also thirty million sheep!

There's always the question, "What is the most beautiful area that you have visited?" This is a very difficult question. This world has so much beauty, and beauty is in the eye of the beholder, so I'm not sure that what I see would be considered the same as what someone else might see. That

171

said, Antarctica would probably head my list, but right along with it, I would have to list Prince Christian Sound off the southern coast of Greenland. It is sixty-six miles of breathtaking splendor. Also the fjords of Norway, the glaciers of Alaska, the Inside Passageway of southern Chile, Milford Sound in southern New Zealand, and some of the bays located on the Marquis Islands in French Polynesia. In our country, the Grand Canyon, Yosemite National Park, and the list goes on and on. As far as buildings are concerned, the Taj Mahal surprised me. In actuality it was so much grander than I had anticipated it to be.

One question that I am often asked, particularly from other doctors, is, "Have you ever been sued?" And the answer is, yes. Three times. However, all three turned out well for me.

The first one occurred way back in 1956 in Muscatine, Iowa. Judy Plank was a patient of mine who was pregnant. She had a lot more nausea and vomiting than we normally expect to see in pregnancy. These episodes of vomiting were associated with upper abdominal pain. We X-rayed her gallbladder right after the birth of the baby and it was full of gallstones. Dr. Swazey decided to go ahead with gallbladder surgery. At the time of surgery, there was uncontrollable bleeding. We only had four units of blood in our little hospital laboratory that were of the same type as Judy's. We gave her all four units but she continued to bleed. Twenty-six miles from Muscatine is Iowa City, which has the University hospital. Dr. Swazey loaded her into an ambulance and went with her to Iowa City, where she was turned over to doctors there. The bleeding had subsided but she became septic and she died four days later. The husband brought a lawsuit against Dr. Swazey for wrongful death and I was included in the suit.

Dr. Peters at that time was the Medical Examiner. I can

remember him coming into the office a couple of weeks later and saying, "I had a Medical Examiner's call last night and it was to the Judy Plank home." It turned out that Mr. Plank had been gone from the house over the weekend, and the pilot light on the furnace had gone out. The furnace leaked gas into his basement. He went into his cold house and attempted to light the pilot light, and there was an explosion, killing Mr. Plank. That was the end of that lawsuit.

The second case occurred in De Pere around 1965. Mrs. Benzschawel worked at the janitorial service at St. Norbert's College. Her regular doctor was Dr. Lenz. When she was at work one day she developed severe abdominal pain with nausea and vomiting and came in to see me because Dr. Lenz was out of town. I thought she was having an acute gallbladder attack and I referred her to Dr. Stoll, a Board Certified Surgeon in Green Bay, and I assisted him as he removed her gallbladder. When the surgery was performed, a drain was left from the gallbladder bed to the outside of her abdomen. When it was time for her to go home, she was continuing to drain. We thought that she could go home and the drain should be left in until the bile drainage stopped. It didn't stop. Two weeks later Dr. Stoll put her back in the hospital, opened her abdomen, took out the drain, and repaired the bile duct region. He thought the bile duct had been injured at the time of surgery, and this accounted for the leak. Dr. Stoll was scheduled for a vacation in the Caribbean and he left two days after surgery. He asked me to continue with her care. Shortly after he left, it became obvious to me that she was continuing to leak bile from the common bile duct. But now there was no drain in place and so it was accumulating inside of her abdomen. I didn't feel that there were any local surgeons who were capable of helping her so I sent her by ambulance to the Mayo Clinic in Rochester, Minnesota. There she had a number of surgical procedures and a number of complications. Then Dr. Stoll and I were served papers for a lawsuit.

My lawyer happened to be a pilot and he wished to get a deposition from the doctor in charge of her care in Rochester. He suggested that Dr. Stoll and I fly with him when he went. We did, and we were flabbergasted when the Mayo doctor pointed at Dr. Stoll and said, "It was all his fault! And I told Mrs. Benzschawel that she should sue you. At the time of our surgery, we found that you had placed a suture around the common bile duct, and furthermore, we have X-rays that we took at the time of surgery that demonstrate this possibility." The case finally came to trial. I was in court all day long for a week, and I tried to take care of my patients during the evening hours. The Mayo doctor testified on tape. When he was asked whether X-rays were taken during the surgery, he said they couldn't be found. When he was questioned about the results of the surgeries she had at Mayo's, he became very defensive. It took a week for Mrs. Benzschawel's lawyers to present all of this material, then it was time for the defense attorney to speak. My lawyer stood up and addressed the judge. He said, "I have sat here for a week now trying to determine with what Dr. Keiser has been charged with doing, and the only thing that they claim that he did was give Mrs. Benzschawel the best physical examination that she had ever had up to that point in her life. And I feel he should be dropped from this suit." Judge Parins called both lawyers up to his desk, and after a short conference, he arose and said, "I agree with the Defense Counsel. Dr. Keiser is no longer part of this litigation." I was there another week and I was on the stand for several hours as Dr. Stoll's defense was presented. In the end, the jury didn't believe the testimony against Dr. Stoll and they found that he was not negligent.

Mrs. Benzschawel's lawyers appealed to the State Supreme Court and they refused to hear it.

During the course of the trial, I had to drop off some things at Dr. Stoll's house. He had previously been in South America on vacation and had an opportunity to purchase a jaguar. The jaguar was a cub, and he had raised it from that point and kept it in his basement as a pet. When I entered his house, he invited me to come downstairs to see his "cat." As I went into the basement, I noticed there was a cabinet along one wall that went almost to the ceiling. Up on the top of this cabinet lay his jaguar. As he saw me, he jumped down from his perch. He did this very easily and quietly. He walked over to me. Dr. Stoll said in a low voice, "Don't move. He just wants to check you out." As he approached me, he raised up on his hind legs, placing one forepaw on each of my shoulders. His face was opposite my face and was only four or five inches away. As he proceeded to lick his lips, Dr. Stoll kept saying, "Don't move now, please don't move." I sure felt like moving, but no way was I going to move! Then he jumped down and returned to his perch up on the cabinet.

The third and last of my lawsuits happened when I was sailing. An elderly gentleman was coming down the stairway from the balcony to the main floor of the show lounge. There was low-level lighting on the edge of the steps and he missed a step and fell about three steps. The next afternoon he came into the infirmary and told me that in his younger days, he was a football player and he had injured his knees on several occasions, and now he believed his knee was dislocated. Before examining his knee, I took him back to get an X-ray. There were no fractures or dislocations—none that I could see, at any rate. He could move his knee, but he had pain, even to touch, on the back of his leg just above his knee. I explained to him that I could see no injuries to the bones. I thought that he had soft tissue injuries that should be evaluated by his own doctor when he got home. There, they could do an MRI and see just how bad his injuries were. In the meantime, he should use a knee brace and return to me anytime that he needed to see me for any reason. The next day he came in and asked for a cane. He said that his balance wasn't very good with a knee brace. I gave him a cane and I didn't see him again during the remaining three days aboard the ship.

He didn't go to his own doctor, as I had instructed him, for two weeks. Then he was told that he had a partial rupture of his quadriceps tendon and that he would need surgery. Shortly after that, I got a call from a lawyer in Seattle saying that HAL was being sued and I was being included in the suit. The lawyer went on to explain that HAL was usually willing to make small settlements to avoid costly court proceedings. He proceeded to talk to me about the case. Then he went on to say that he didn't feel that settling this case was appropriate, and that he was going to ask for a jury trial if it was okay with me. I agreed. He said that the suit was proceeding in Seattle and that he would have to have the plaintiff come from his home in Chicago to Seattle for a deposition—but it would not be necessary for me to come to Seattle. This was in January, and he said, "I'll take your deposition in Florida. By the way, how's the weather right now?" I told him this time of the year the weather is always good in Florida.

The plaintiff hadn't thought about going to Seattle. He had figured we would just come up with a little money and that would be all there was to it. His lawyer approached mine with an offer to settle for $5,000. We refused. Then he lowered it to $1,000 and my lawyer set a date for when they had to be in Seattle for a deposition. The plaintiff refused to go to Seattle; the case was dropped. Lawsuits are always traumatic. They're always time consuming. And even when they turn out as these three cases did, they are no fun at all!

One last question I get is, "What type of people go on cruises?" There are three general categories of passengers that we see on board and they are: the newlyweds, the overfeds, and the nearly deads. I am of course being facetious. However, HAL does cater to the older population and to the handicapped. We have staterooms that have wider front doors for wheelchair access and also wider doors to the bathrooms to make them easily accessible to the handicapped. We have cruises that have dialysis on board, with a special doctor and nursing staff who supervise dialysis only. My nurses and I take care of the general health needs of the dialysis patients. And of course, there are some children and youth on every cruise.

For several years I had been sailing a total of six months out of each year. Last year I was on the water only five months, and this year, 2003, it looks like I will be going out a little less than three months.

What about next year? I had begun to think seriously about retiring. My daughter called and said, "Before you retire, you really should take your grandchildren and your children to Alaska." The Wish List for 2004 came out and I found myself picking voyages not only to Alaska, but to the Amazon River, too. And then, as I looked through the Wish List, I began to think it would be nice to spend a few weeks on the Mediterranean next summer. So will next year, 2004, be my last year sailing? I'm not sure, but if it is, I just may change directions and look for something new to do.

As I look over the story of my life, I wonder, is there some moral in the story? Is there something that can be learned from it? I think so. And to me, this would be that it is never too late in life to make changes.

This September 26, 2003, I will be going to lunch in Madison, Wisconsin. The lunch will be hosted by the State Medical Society for doctors who have been practicing for fifty years. I don't know how many doctors will be there. Yet I do know that I will be honored to be in that group. It has been fifty wonderful years and I feel that I have been truly blessed!

Postscript

When I think of getting old, it is always someone else who comes to my mind. Although I must admit that getting up on the roof to clean out my gutters this spring was just a little more difficult. I hate to think that my next birthday will be my seventy-eighth. Nearly a year has gone by since that dark and stormy night when I lay in my bed thinking about my life. It has been fun to reflect, and it has been rewarding to me and hopefully to others, as I find myself still sailing, and still seeing patients—and still asking the question, "How can I help you?"